Baby Boomers

Can My Eighties Be Like My Fifties?

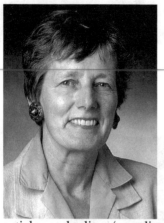

M. Joanna Mellor, DSW, is Assistant Professor at the Wurzweiler School of Social Work, Yeshiva University, New York. Prior to this appointment, Dr. Mellor was Vice President for Information Services at Lighthouse International, Assistant Professor in the Department of Geriatrics and Adult Development, Mount Sinai Medical Center, and Executive Director of the Hunter/Mount Sinai Geriatric Education Center. She has been an Adjunct Instructor at the Hunter School of Social Work since 1984. Dr. Mellor is author of several articles and editor/co-editor of five books, including *Special Aging Populations and Systems Linkages* and *Advancing Gerontological Social Work Education.* She is co-editor of the *Journal of Gerontological Social Work* and a past president of the State Society of Aging of New York.

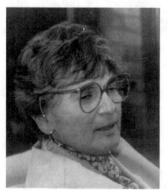

Helen Rehr, DSW, D.Sc.(Hon), is currently Professor of Community Medicine Emerita and Consultant on social-health research, education, and program planning to Mount Sinai School of Medicine and Medical Center. She is the retired Director, Department of Social Work Services, the Director of the academic Division of Social Work, and Director of the Division of Continuous Education of the Brookdale Center of Mount Sinai. She has been active internationally in Israel and Australia, where she has held visiting professorships. Dr. Rehr is the author, co-author, and editor of more than a hundred published studies, reports, articles, chapters, and books and the recipient of numerous honors, including Distinguished Social Work Practitioner for the National Academies of Practice, the Knee-Wittman Award for Lifetime Achievement, and the Ida M. Cannon Award of the Society of Hospital Social Work Directors, the American Hospital Association, and has been inducted into the Hall of Fame of both Hunter and Columbia. Although retired from Mount Sinai in 1986, she remains active at the institution and in a number of professional and community organizations.

Baby Boomers

Can My Eighties Be Like My Fifties?

M. Joanna Mellor, DSW
Helen Rehr, DSW, Editors

 Springer Publishing Company

 Lifestyles and Issues in Aging Series

Without the contribution of over 300 participants, the majority of whom were Baby Boomers and health care professionals (many of whom were Baby Boomers as well) at the three Summit Series, this book would not be possible. We believe the many issues raised should set the parameters for deliberations by Baby Boomers for their future social and health wants and needs.

Springer Publishing Company, Inc.
11 West 42nd Street, 15th Floor
New York, NY 10036-8022

Acquisitions Editor: Helvi Gold
Production Editor: Jeanne Libby
Cover design by Joanne Honigman

05 06 07 08 09 / 5 4 3 2 1

Library of Congress Cataloging-in-Publication Data

Mellor, M. Joanna.
  Baby boomers : can my eighties be like my fifties / M. Joanna Mellor and Helen Rehr.—1st ed.
      p. ; cm. — (Springer series on lifestyles and issues in aging)
  Includes bibliographical references and index.
  Summary: "Based on a conference funded by the Robert Wood Johnson Foundation, this book brings together baby boomers and health care professionals to explore baby boomers' perceptions of their future social-health care expectations and needs"—Provided by publisher.
  ISBN 0-8261-2615-4 (soft cover)
  1. Baby boom generation—Health and hygiene—United States—Congresses. 2. Baby boom generation—United States—Psychology—Congresses. 3. Baby boom generation—Retirement—United States—Congresses. 4. Baby boom generation—United States—Social conditions—21th century—Congresses. 5. Health attitudes—Age factors—United States—Congresses. 6. Health behavior—Age factors—United States—Congresses. 7. Medical care—Needs assessment—United States—Congresses. 8. Medical care—United States—Forecasting—Congresses. I. Rehr, Helen. II. Title. III. Series: Springer series on life styles and issues in aging. [DNLM: 1. Needs Assessment—trends—Aged—Congresses. 2. Needs Assessment—trends—Middle Aged—Congresses. 3. Attitude to Health—Aged—Congresses. 4. Attitude to Health—Middle Aged—Congresses. WT 100 M527b 2005]
RA408.B33M455 2005
613'.0438—dc22   2005005889

Printed in the United States of America by Maple-Vail Book Manufacturing Group.

Contents

Contributors		*vii*
Foreword by Jeanette Takamura		*ix*
Preface by Rose Dobrof		*xiii*
Acknowledgment		*xv*

1	Introduction: An Unsuspecting Future *Helen Rehr*	1
2	Overview: Current Seniors, Baby Boomers, Minorities, and Health Disparities	8
3	A Baby Boomer's Perception of the Baby Boom Era *Sue Woodman*	27
4	Income Security: Social Security, Work, Pensions, and Savings	35
5	Health Care Security: Medicare, Medicaid, Health Insurance, and Health Care Delivery	46
6	Long-Term Care: Who Will Care for Us?	60
7	End-of-Life-Care *Karen O. Kaplan*	74
8	Retirement, Lifestyles, and Roles: Leisure, Volunteering, and Work	84
9	Living Arrangements	97

10 Aging in Place: 111
   ~~Shaping Communities for Tomorrow's Baby~~
   Boomers—
   Naturally Occurring Retirement Communities
   (NORCs)
   Fredda Vladeck

11 Health Care Professionals and Their Education 123

12 Community Collaboration and Advocacy 145

13 *Can* My Eighties Be Like My Fifties?: 158
   Conclusions and Recommendations

Appendix 173

Appendix I   Social Work Fellows Planning Committee 181

Appendix II   Summit Presenters 182

Appendix III   Workshop Leaders and Reporters 185

Index *187*

Contributors

Karen Orloff Kaplan, MPH, ScD, is President and CEO of Partnership for Caring, America's Voices for the Dying (PfC) and National Program Director of Last Acts. Before her appointment at PfC, Dr. Kaplan served as Executive Director of Choice in Dying, Inc., a non-profit organization known for its advocacy on behalf of dying people and their loved ones. She was the founding Executive Director of the National Center for Social Policy and Practice, the research and policy arm of the 140,000-member National Association of Social Workers. Dr. Kaplan also served as a health staff associate to Rep. Ron Wyden (D-Oregon), advising him about health and social issues, particularly as they related to older persons.

Fredda Vladeck, CSW, is director of the Aging in Place Initiative of the United Hospital Fund and the founding Director of the first comprehensive Naturally Occurring Retirement Community (NORC), a nationally recognized model program of supportive services for older persons aging in place. Ms. Vladeck spent five years in Washington, DC, as Advisor for Aging and Health Policy to the President of the International Brotherhood of Teamsters and then as Director of Health Policy for the National Council of Senior Citizens, before returning to New York and taking up her current position.

Sue Woodman is a freelance writer specializing in health and social issues. She has written widely for U.S. and British publications, most recently, *My Generation*, an AARP magazine for baby boomers. She is the author of *Last Rights: The Struggle over the Right to Die*. Ms. Woodman's presentation at the 4/02 Summit is published as chapter 3 in this book.

Foreword

D istinctively high fertility rates during the 1946–1964 post-World War II years resulted in an unprecedented upsurge in the nation's population. As a group, the seventy-six million Baby Boomers born during this period have tested many of our deeply rooted social values, beliefs, and institutions, and have redefined our sociocultural norms. The traditional definition of the family, gender roles, sexual orientations, and racial and ethnic biases are among the social institutions and phenomena that were challenged by members of this generational cohort. The marketplace has also been shaped with the developmental needs, productive and leisure activities, and consumer preferences of the Boomers and their parents.

Beginning in 2011, the leading edge of the Baby Boom generation will celebrate their 65th birthdays. They will come of age in a nation with a growing number of older persons, many of whom will be able to enjoy the gift of longevity. Many will achieve the status of centenarians in the future. Many more will represent one of several generations of older persons within an increasing number of families. However, longevity is not a privilege limited to persons and families in the United States or in the developed world. In 2011, the number of Baby Boomers in the U.S. will exceed twice the total population of Canada. By the second half of this century, the older American population of 84.5 million will seem relatively small when compared to the 331 million older persons in China, who will nearly equal the total projected population of persons of all ages in the U.S.

Often portrayed as monolithic and miscast as homogeneous, Boomers will become older Americans over a period of two decades (2011–2029). Those born in 1946 include former President Bill Clinton, current President George W. Bush, developer Donald Trump, and actor Diane Keaton. These Boomers were born in the year in which the first meeting of the United Nations was held on Long Island and in which the World War II War Crimes trials began. In contrast, those born in 1964—eighteen years later and at the tail end of the Boomer genera-tion—include Olympian Bonnie Blair and actors Keanu Reeves and Calista Flockhart. The Civil Rights Act was signed into law, the Warren Commission Report was published, Nelson Mandela was sentenced to life in prison, and the War on Poverty was declared in 1964. One could argue that the leading edge and the tail end Boomers are more different than alike.

Unlike preceding generations, the majority of Boomers have grown up as beneficiaries of significantly improved public health and education systems. They have lived through years in which the economy was ex-panding and flourishing. At the start of the twenty-first century, they enjoyed a national mood that was relatively optimistic. They can claim better health and more years of education as a group. They have not been immune, however, from income and health disparities. As is the case today, single, minority, elderly women living alone who earn less than two wage-earner families or other older Americans will have less discretionary income, be less able to save, and be most at risk of impover-ishment. At least one study has predicted that income disparities will differentiate Baby Boomers from each other, irrespective of gender, and cause those at the lower end of the socioeconomic scale to remain in the workplace well past age 65. In fact, many Baby Boomers, like older Americans of earlier generations, may have only their monthly Social Security check upon which to rely for their retirement income. This will be the case for those similar to the Baby Boomers who, a 2000 poll found, could not save sufficiently for their advanced years (Heinz Foundation, 2000). The implications of this are many, particularly in light of the anticipated discussion of the future of Social Security. Unfor-tunately, as chapter 4 suggests, the extent to which Social Security monthly benefits prevent poverty among near-poor elderly Americans and the pervasiveness of financial illiteracy in our populace, irrespective of age, are not widely understood.

It is no secret that the incidence of most chronic illnesses tends to be higher in racial and ethnic minority populations. Although it is encouraging that evidence-based care is becoming more prevalent be-cause systematic reviews of randomized clinical trials and the translation and transfer of research findings are more commonplace, study samples have not tended to include an adequate number of minority partici-pants. Thus, health care professionals cannot count upon reliable find-ings from empirical research applicable to these individuals. Without culturally sensitive, evidence-based care provided by culturally competent professionals, and without adequate, affordable health insurance coverage, minority older Boomers cannot expect health care access and quality to be at acceptable levels.

As they age, Boomers may be expected to establish new roles for older adults that assume reliance upon technology and on-demand access to information. These roles will inevitably reflect the cohort's diversity—more pronounced when additional foreign-born Boomers are added to the mix. Pioneering Baby Boomers will determine and help to legitimate a rich spectrum of options if they are bold in the application of their expertise, experience, time, and energy as older workers and volunteers. Observing less civic engagement (i.e., voting and joining community groups) among Boomers than among their parents, the Harvard School of Public Health study, "Reinventing Aging: Baby Boomers and Civic Engagement," investigated whether Boomers can be engaged and whether civic organizations will be prepared for their participation. The study recognized the extent to which civic engagement and role redefinition can be influenced and moved along by concerted social marketing by the communications and entertainment industries. The report also noted the need to urge Boomers to plan for their later years so that their lives then might be meaningful and satisfying.

Given the sum total of their impact over decades past, we can reasonably anticipate that Boomers will not simply age. They will determine how we in the United States and in the global community will perceive and treat older adults and aging as a process. There is evidence already that persons of all ages do not define being "old" chronologically, but rather by whether one has disabling physical or mental limitations (NCOA, 2000). With this the case, the Boomers are likely to express new standards for quality of life in the later years. Although we must wait to see what emerges over the long term, the New York Academy of Medicine and its partnering sponsors of the Summit Series on Baby Boomers have already tapped into indications that Boomers do not want their parents' lifestyles for themselves in their older years.

This book for health professionals examines and discusses an impressive array of social and health concerns that are of immediate value to our Boomers and all who will care for them. It urges timely attention to and the reform of social and health policies and systems that have remained tied to outdated premises—many adopted in the last half of the twentieth century in response to the needs and interests of youthful

Baby Boomers and their parents. The book offers a clear view of knowledge and skills that must be acquired by each professional in order that the aging Boomer population might be served effectively. It provides a clarion call to the health care professions and it illumines essential components of the programs and services that will be needed by the Boomers, a cohort that is nearly twice as large as the 46 million-person Generation X born between 1963 and 1974. It also draws from the rich experiences and scholarship of leading gerontologists and geriatricians who have generously contributed their rich familiarity with national and New York City developments and innovations, among them, for example, Naturally Occurring Retirement Communities (NORCs). For this comprehensive, rich resource on a segment of our population that will inevitably shape the twenty-first century, Dr. Helen Rehr and her colleagues must be commended.

U.S. Department of Labor. (1997). *The aging baby boom: Implications for employment and training program.* Washington, D.C.: The Urban Institute.

Jeanette C. Takamura, MSW, PhD
Dean, Columbia University School of Social Work

Preface

The genesis of this publication lies with Dr. Helen Rehr, Professor Emerita of Mount Sinai School of Medicine who, as we entered the twenty-first century, expressed concern that hospitals, home care agencies, and other social service agencies in the social service health and aging networks might not be prepared for the aging of the Baby Boom generation and its utilization of services. Dr. Rehr, Patricia Volland, Associate Director, Dr. Nadine Gartrell, Program Officer, and the Social Work Section of the New York Academy of Medicine joined forces to plan a series of Summit Meetings designed to develop a guide for social workers and health care professionals concerned about social-health needs and delivery systems for Baby Boomers as they age. That was 2001; now, as I write this, it is 2004, and this publication, *Baby Boomers: Can My Eighties Be Like My Fifties?*, is one of the fruits of those Summit Meetings.

The Baby Boomers are fast coming to our attention as the caregiving generation for their functionally dependent parents. They have now reached maturity, with the leading edge of the generation in their mid-fifties. In 2011, they will be observing their 65th birthdays and, to use Dr. Robert Butler's wonderful phrase, "the Baby Boom generation will go to the Golden Pond." By the year 2029, the youngest boomers will have reached 65 years of age and millions will be over 85. In 2001, looking ahead to the Summit Meetings, I asked, in the *Journal of Gerontological Social Work* (Vol. 35, No.1), will the Baby Boomers "with a higher percentage of never married and divorced and/or childless people in the generation be more likely to utilize the services of our institutions and agencies? What kind of clients/patients will they be, assertive or compliant, for instance? In the absence of large family networks, will Baby Boomers depend on the kindness of friends and neighbors, if chronic illness and disability become their fate in their later years? What kind of relationship will they want with the professionals to whom they come for help?"

The questions I raised and many more were topics of discussion at the three Summit Meetings, which included keynote presentations from several eminent leaders in health and social services, followed by workshop discussions by Baby Boomers and social/health service providers. I have just finished reading the 13 chapters of this publication based on the presentations and discussions. It offers a marvelously drawn picture of the Baby Boomers from a variety of perspectives and vantage points, and my prediction is that this will be a much used and much cited text. Congratulations are due to Helen, Pat, Nadine, and the Social Work Fellows of the New York Academy of Medicine who planned and organized the Summit Meetings; to Joanna who did such a superb job of writing and editing; to the guest authors who contributed and shared their special expertise; and to all those who participated as presenters and discussants.

Rose Dobrof, DSW
Brookdale Professor of Gerontology, Hunter College

Acknowledgment

The editors and Social Work Fellows of the New York Academy of Medicine wish to acknowledge the support of the Robert Wood Johnson Foundation for the three Summit Series, "Can My Eighties Be Like My Fifties?" held at the Academy, October 2001 through October 2002, for invited Baby Boomers and health care professionals. In addition, they are indebted to the following for sponsorship of the summit series:

The New York Academy of Medicine
Mount Sinai Medical Center
Brookdale Center on Aging of Hunter College
The International Longevity Center
AARP

The Social Work Fellows of The New York Academy of Medicine (Appendix I) planned and implemented the summit series with the invaluable assistance of Dr. Nadine Gartrell of the Academy. They are especially indebted for the wonderful presentations of Drs. Robert Butler, Bruce Vladeck, Donna Shalala, John Rother, Ron Adelman, Michael Diaz, Mathy Mezey, Katherine Briar-Lawson, and to the journalist, Sue Woodman (Appendix II). The series would not have been so successful without the contributions of the leaders and recorders of the workshops (Appendix III)—but most of all that made by the participant Baby Boomers and health care professionals. It is all of their efforts and the generous support of the Jayne Silberman Fund that have made this publication possible.

Chapter 1

Introduction:
An Unsuspecting Future

Helen Rehr

"We must age but do we have to grow old?" was the question Dr. Donna Shalala introduced in her presentation at the Third Summit Meeting on the Baby Boomers' perception of their aging.

Over a period of 18 months in three sessions, Baby Boomers and health care professionals deliberated on their perceptions of the future of the Baby Boomers as they age. The meetings took place on October 10, 2001, April 24, 2002, and October 25, 2002. The invited participants were Baby Boomers, health care social workers, nurses and doctors who were practitioners and educators, and a few political officials. The objectives of the series were (1) to identify Baby Boomers' perceptions of their future social and health care expectations, needs, and wants, (2) to increase Baby Boomers' and health care professionals' awareness of projected demographic and social changes in society, and (3) to encourage Baby Boomers, providers, educators, and politicians to think proactively about tomorrow's anticipated needs.

The summit series, titled "Can My Eighties Be Like My Fifties?" was planned by the Social Work Fellows of the New York Academy of Medicine with the support of the Robert Wood Johnson Foundation. The

Fellows, many of whom have worked with the elderly, recognized from their experiences and studies that current knowledge and services are related to today's elderly and not tomorrow's. They were prompted by a concern that the Baby Boomer generation, many of whose members are now in their fifties, may be unprepared for the future.

The subject for the series became a reality as the Social Work Fellows were joined by the leaders of the Brookdale Center on Aging (Hunter College), the International Longevity Center, the Geriatric Education Center, the Mount Sinai Medical Center, and the American Association of Retired Persons (AARP), as all agreed the fields of gerontology and geriatrics were committed to enhancing services for today's elderly. They believed it was time to deliberate on social and health policies and services for the future.

The initial summit meeting brought together over 100 Baby Boomers and health and social work service providers and educators. Over the three summits, more than 340 people participated and made their thoughts known. They learned that there were over 75 million Baby Boomers currently on the scene and that they would be the largest generation ever to reach 65 and over between 2010 and 2030.

In less than 20 years, more than 20% of the United States population will be over 65 years of age, doubling today's number. There are greater differences and more diversity within this Baby Boomer group than in their parents' and grandparents' groups. Today the minorities—blacks and Hispanics—face even a greater difference from whites in their poorer health status, income levels, access to care, insurance coverage, and life expectancy. By 2030, there will be almost nine million people over 85 years of age. Although the forecasts for health and financial security are relatively positive, it is projected that the majority of the future elderly will need some level of social and health care. Also, unless there is a cure for Alzheimer's disease, it is anticipated that 20% will suffer from that disease and/or mental illness. Malignancies, cardiovascular and cerebrovascular diseases, orthopedic and cognitive impairments are expected to persist, with concomitant physical and social limitations.

The first meeting of the series took place shortly following the attack on the World Trade Center. Participants' early responses, which reflected anxiety and uncertainty about their future, may have been colored by the significance of that tragic event. As the Baby Boomers talked about themselves, they told the professionals that the way their parents lived was not for them! Although they appreciated the help of the social service and health care professionals in assisting their parents with their needs, and thus themselves, their parents' life patterns were not what they wanted. "We don't want to face what our elderly parents are facing today. Aging will be different for us." They believe that present-day gerontological experts are helpful, but that they are dealing with twentieth-century needs of the aging, whereas their future will be different. The Baby Boomers described their parents with their chronic illnesses and limitations as needing to draw on nursing homes, assisted living, or caretakers in their homes and/or residential homes to meet their needs.

The Baby Boomers noted that "old age is not for me." They did not see aging as their concern, agreeing with Dr. Shalala that they may age, but they would not get old. Their view was more along Sue Woodman's thinking that today's Baby Boomers believe they will sustain their youth. They focus, if they do it at all, on anti-aging medicine. When they think of aging, again if they think of it at all, it is not about growing old but rather in terms of wellness, independence, and self-sufficiency.

This group of Baby Boomers described themselves and current situations, in response to surveys:

- In caring for their parents, most thought the health care services were poor or fair, and the social services were somewhat better, citing these as fair.
- Their own health status was good; they use the Internet and media to become informed about any symptoms they may have. They do not rely as much on professional services as their parents do but will use them to follow up on their needs.
- They hoped to be able to retire before they were 70, but the majority thought they would need to work longer to secure their financial future before retiring.
- If long-term care should be needed, they expected it would be via self-pay, and were doubtful that it would be an employer contribution, as that benefit seems to be disappearing.
- They will not be living with their children, but in their own homes with partners, they hope, and they believe they will have access to friends and relatives.
- If they need help to live at home, they want it to be available and affordable.
- They do not think of end-of-life planning although a number of this group has completed advance directives and health care proxies.
- They see their future more in a social and environmental context than in a medical one, but they believe that maintenance is key to staying healthy.

The group of Baby Boomers also cited a number of beliefs and concerns:

- They do not expect their children to care for them, nor do they want them to have the burden of responsibility as they themselves have for their aging and frail parents.
- They do not believe their children will be nearby anyway, as their children are quite mobile.
- They dislike the negative stereotypes of the elderly and aging portrayed in public arenas; they think these depictions may have contributed to today's ageism.
- They do not see serious illness in their future.
- They think Medicare and Social Security will be negatively altered, and there are uncertainties for the future; self-pay will be more the norm.
- They are dissatisfied with the current health care system; costs keep rising and they fear the implications of the commercialization of health care and its impact on them.
- They want living arrangements that support quality of life.
- They are uncertain about the future status of their pensions and of their employer–employee health insurance.
- They criticize the Administration's policy on immigration, believing that it will curtail a labor force of home aides and other health care workers, making at-home help not as available to them as it is to their parents.

The Baby Boomers did have a "wish list" as they voiced their expectations for their future. They were clear on wanting good health, economic security, quality and affordable housing, family proximity or accessibility, good relationships with their family, and a network of friends. They saw themselves as mobile and independent, wanting to remain active and to have leisure opportunities. They would prefer to live in intergenerational communities, with good support services, if needed, from trained and understanding help. Quality medical, mental health and social services should be available and affordable.

In the main, Baby Boomers describe feeling good about their relationships with family and friends. They are supportive of their elderly parents; they consider themselves in fairly good shape emotionally and spiritually. They believe they will be able to cope and to have a successful aging.

What surfaced from the three summit meetings were a host of probabilities that both Baby Boomers and health care professionals need to consider now for tomorrow:

- Baby Boomers will increase in numbers.
- They will begin to retire in 2008 when the oldest will be 62.
- They will live longer than their parents did.
- More will be single, and those who are married will have fewer children.
- More will be wealthier, but there will be a sizable vulnerable population of low-income individuals.
- Baby Boomers are not a homogeneous group; there are more disparities and more diversity in wealth and health.
- Chronic illness and disability will not have been eradicated; Baby Boomers will still need to understand disease/illness, but both Baby Boomers and health care professionals will need to concentrate on functional and psychological effects of illness and disability.
- Today's health care professionals relate to today's elderly needs, and are educated in that context, rather than preparing for future needs.
- The commercialization of health delivery needs to be reviewed for tomorrow's needs.
- The current financial crisis in health care delivery affects service availability.
- Today's medical model needs to be rethought in a more comprehensive social–health model of care.
- Changes in Medicare and Social Security may produce more elderly at risk for health care and financial stability problems.
- Shortages in health care professionals, particularly nurses, social workers, and support staff, will affect the availability of adequate care.
- Baby Boomers' tend to use the Internet without professional consultation.
- Health education and prevention are inadequate today.
- Collaboration among the health care professions needs to be taught and enhanced.
- Continuing education for health care providers should be mandated.
- Partnership concepts between patients and health care providers need to be developed.
- Studies for best practice and programs are needed.

Even as the participants expressed the uncertainties affecting the economy, their concerns with the health care system, with social welfare for many, and with their hyperkinetic lifestyles, the prediction for Baby Boomers is that they will live longer, live better, and be healthier than their parents. Even ageism, the stereotyping of the elderly, was forecast as on the wane and will probably no longer be a public bias when they reach their sixty-fifth year. They did face concerns for those who will not have it "better." They acknowledged that there will be those who will be chronically ill and will need financial assistance and a range of social–health services and supports, and for this group, and perhaps for the majority of Baby Boomers, today's social–health care inequality needs to be dealt with. As they view retirement, leisure, and self-fulfillment, these are their projections:

- Community-based care is most desirable.
- Holding onto youthful interests and securing new ones will help in "not growing old."
- Autonomy in selection of services and providers is strongly preferred, individual choice is critical, and government should offer opportunities for enhanced services.
- Biogenetic aspects of aging and how to maximize them are most important.
- The individual has self-responsibility as to his/her human life course.

The conclusion of the participants in the series supported the initial remarks of Dr. Robert Butler, who opened the summit sessions, with "Society is unprepared for longevity." There are changes occurring in health care, its delivery, in governmental programs, in industry's benefit programs, and in private support systems. Market forces are transforming health, social, and economic resources. We can expect remarkable biotechnical innovations. Technology and Medicare changes will result in a longer life span, it is hoped with a good quality of life expectation. The conclusion of the sessions (see chapter 13) reflected the need to activate Baby Boomers and public and health care providers to the issues they will face tomorrow. Given their expressed projections for the future, Baby Boomers and health care professionals saw the benefit in joining in a coalition to inform themselves for tomorrow's needs, and to secure and support the provision of human social–health resources. R. D. Putnam (2000) suggests that the 9/11 episode may have changed us. He believes we are more "we." A communitarianism may be developing. He advises that we should "seize the moment to go together."

The presentations and workshop discussions were audiotaped. The initial plan was to publish the series in edited proceedings. However, the Social Work Fellows of the New York Academy of Medicine concluded that two publications dealing with the summit content were preferable: this publication, detailing the presentations and workshop deliberations for the academic and provider communities as well as for Baby Boomers, and a briefer publication for Baby Boomers and the general public.

This book is addressed to the health care professionals in the fields of geriatrics and gerontology. The Social Work Section of the New York Academy of Medicine is indebted to the Jayne M. Silberman Fund for its support. The second publication (in preparation) will address the Baby Boomers, the first of whom will reach the age of 65 by 2011.

The question; "Can My Eighties Be Like My Fifties?" will require Baby Boomers and social–health care professionals to find ways to continue the discussions on their beliefs, expectations, and projections that were initiated by the summit series.

REFERENCE

Putnam, R. D. (2000). *Bowling alone.* New York: Simon & Schuster.

Chapter 2

Overview: Current Seniors, Baby Boomers, Minorities, and Health Disparities

U.S. SENIORS TODAY

Twelve and a half percent (12.5%) of the U.S. population is 65 years or older.

Thirty five million persons are 65 years of age or older.

Sixty-eight thousand persons are 100 years or older.

Four and a half percent (4.5%) of older persons are in institutional care at any given time.

One third of those living in the community live alone.

Over 60% of persons over the age of 80 live independently.

Sixteen percent (16%) are minority elderly.

Twelve percent (12%) are at or below the poverty line.

One third of those over 75 years of age are at or below the poverty level.

Two thirds rate their health as excellent, very good, or good.

One third report that they are handicapped from one or more chronic conditions.

Four and a half million persons over 65 have a mental illness.

Approximately 5% of those over 65 years and living in the community are diagnosed with major depression and another 15% have significant depressive symptoms that are substantially disabling.

Medicare recipients spend 50% of their income out of pocket for health care.

Over 50% of Medicare funds are spent in medical care of the last six months of life.

Less than 10% of older adults have long term care insurance policies.

BABY BOOMERS TOMORROW

On May 19, 2011, the oldest Baby Boomers will turn 65 years of age.

By 2030, twenty percent (20%) of the U.S. population will be 65 years or older.

By 2030, 76 million persons in the U.S. will be 65 years or older.

Sixty-nine to seventy (69–70) million Baby Boomers will survive to age 65.

By 2030, there will be 8.9 million persons over 85 years of age.

By 2050, there will be 835,000 persons over the age of 100.

Fifty percent (50%) of those over 85 will need some level of social and health care assistance.

By 2030, 25% will be minority elderly.

By 2030, more than 9 million persons over the age of 65 will have a mental illness.

By 2040, 14 million persons will be suffering from Alzheimer's disease.

Sixty percent (60%) will be living independently but alone.

Fifty-seven percent (57%) of Baby Boomers are concerned that they will not have sufficient income in retirement.

Medicare costs will increase from 2% to 6% of the Gross National Product between now and 2040.

Social Security outlays to recipients will increase by 50–100% between now and 2040.*

---

*Source: The above statistics are taken from the U.S. Census website and from the Administration on Aging website, including the 2000 U.S. Census.

THE BABY BOOMERS: WHO ARE THEY AND
WHO WILL THEY BECOME?

> Can my eighties be like my fifties? No, not likely. It's a very
> different stage of life, a different style of life.
>
> Robert Butler

The fact is indisputable. In the middle of the last century, the U.S. experienced a sudden surge in births, resulting in a generation that outnumbered all preceding generations and has not been equaled since. This generation of babies, born between 1946 and 1964, has become popularly known as the Baby Boom generation or Baby Boomers. Each generation leaves its mark, but the sheer number of Baby Boomers—76 million—has impacted on U.S. society at every stage of their lives in a manner that is unprecedented.

Now in their middle years, who and what are the Baby Boomers of today? And, more importantly for those who believe in sound social planning and the future, what will the Baby Boom generation be like when it reaches old age? The leading edge of the generation will reach 65 years of age on May, 19, 2011. Will the Baby Boomers be ready for their old age and will the United States be prepared for the great numbers of elderly?

BABY BOOMERS TODAY

The 76 million Baby Boomers, born just after World War II, in an era of economic growth, came of age in the sixties and are now in their young-middle years, aged 38 to 57. Although raising fewer children than their parents, they are more likely to experience both divorce and remarriage as well as a greater number of job changes during their working years. It is a diverse population. The front-running Baby Boomers and those born at the tail end of the nineteen-year spread are almost two decades apart and tend to have differing experiences, attitudes, and expectations. In addition to this diversity, there is variety of ethnicity, cultures, and socioeconomic levels, as well as a growing number of foreign-born persons. There are more Baby Boomers living in cities and suburbia than in rural areas. All these differences make it impossible to arrive at a composite Baby Boomer who represents this generation. In looking toward the future, our tendency is to homogenize the Baby

Boomers but it is essential that we simultaneously recognize the extent of the differences among them. As Cutler (1998) remarks, "the texture and magnitude of boomer diversity are just as important as the magnitude of their demographic numbers."

It is frequently supposed that Baby Boomers are comfortably well off, but income levels vary considerably. A 1996 poll found that more (57%) of the Baby Boomers surveyed were concerned that they would not have sufficient income in their retirement years than those (43%) who were confident that they will (Cutler, 1998).

Concern related to insufficient income in the future is possibly fueled by the fact that Baby Boomers judge both Social Security and Medicare as programs at risk. Their support for these programs is higher than the confidence they hold in them (AARP, 1999). This uncertainty about the viability of our federal income and health insurance programs comes at a time when companies are cutting back on the retirement benefits and health insurance offered to their employees. Costs are being shifted from the employers to the employees themselves. Even before the recent downturn in the U.S. economy, an increasing number of those aged 50 to 64 years were uninsured, with fewer employers offering health care coverage to early retirees. In addition, private health insurance covered fewer people in 1999 than ten years earlier in 1989.

The Baby Boomers are in better health than their parents were at the same age. This population uses health services to a greater degree than their parents did, receives more vaccinations and screenings, and includes fewer smokers. The incidences of heart disease, stroke, and limitations in physical functioning have all declined. However, it is disturbing to note that the American generation with the highest proportion of overweight and obesity is the Baby Boom generation. Sixty-eight percent of Baby Boomers are considered to be over their ideal weight. Equally disturbing is the fact that the majority (70%) of those over 50 are living with at least one chronic health condition.

On the plus side, studies indicate that as a generation, Baby Boomers are psychologically resilient and better informed than their parents' generation. They are "more skeptical, have higher expectations, and are more proactive consumers of health care than those over 65" (AARP, 2002). They are also more likely to use alternative/complementary medicine, seeking information from the Internet and the media and utilizing it. Both of these practices, although a welcome sign that Baby Boomers are taking an active role in their health care, need to be accompanied by a warning. Not all alternative medical practices are effective, and many of the recommended herbal remedies and much of the anti-aging medicine and therapies are of little use and may even be harmful. Similarly, health and medical information gleaned from the Internet is not always accurate or complete. Seekers of health information are advised to limit their searches to the websites of academic institutions, medical associations, government agencies, and health advocacy groups and be cautious of the information on other sites. Former Surgeon General Dr. Everett Koop strongly advises on his website, "Be sure to see a doctor. The Internet allows patients to make decisions in tandem with their doctor to get better outcomes" (Koop, E., www.drkoop.com). Baby Boomers and others need advice from health care professionals before they utilize the remedies and information they acquire.

In observing the current health status of the Baby Boom generation, it is important to recognize the marked health disparities that currently exist between white non-Hispanics and members of minority populations. The future U.S. older population promises to be much more racially and ethnically diverse than today's elders and we must anticipate increased strain on our health care systems unless we, as a society, succeed now in reducing the disparities in health care.

MINORITY HEALTH: DISPARITIES AND ISSUES

Introduction

There is well-documented and compelling evidence that the health of minority populations in the U.S. lags behind that of U.S. whites. This is true in nearly all areas: higher rates of cancer, heart disease, and diabetes; less access to appropriate health care; poorer outcomes from treatment; lower level of health in general; and lower life expectancy. Compared with today's older population, the Baby Boomers include a higher percentage of minority persons and as a group they rate health issues (37%) higher than economic issues (31%) as a concern for themselves and their families (AARP, 2001). If the health disparities continue to exist in the years ahead, the combination of greater numbers of older persons and an increased percentage of minority persons among them is likely to adversely impact the quality of life of older Baby Boomers and place an increased burden on the health care system.

For instance, African Americans experience more years living with chronic health problems than their white counterparts (Crimmins & Saito, 2001).

The federal government and health care providers have been aware of these disparities in health and health care for many years and the Federal government has long been interested in righting the inequalities. In the mid-eighties, the U.S. Department of Health and Human Services established a Task Force on Black and Minority Health. The Task Force found wide disparities between minorities and whites in all age groups and noted in its report a "continuing disparity of death and illness experienced by Blacks and other minority Americans as compared with our nation's population as a whole" (U.S. Department of Health and Human Services, 1985). There now exists a National Center on Minority Health and Health Disparities with a mission to promote minority health and to reduce and eliminate health disparities.

Health Disparities: The Evidence

Health disparities between minorities and whites exist in all areas, from incidence of disease to access to care and treatment and outcomes.

Health Status

Whereas 10% of whites report that they are in only fair or poor health, 16% of blacks and 17% of Hispanics report being in fair or poor health (Agency for Healthcare, Research and Quality, 2003). This is to be expected, given the higher rate of illness among minorities. Cancer death rates among African Americans, both men and women, are approximately 35% higher than for white women. The incidence of lung cancer among black men in the U.S. is at a high of 117 per 100,000, and that of prostate cancer is the highest in the world at 180.6 per 100,000. Although the incidence among white men is also quite high, it is distinctly lower than among blacks (AHRQ, 2003).

The life expectancy for minority women is five years less than for whites, and health disparities even appear to be increasing in some areas (AHRQ website). The most compelling health issues facing minority women are cancer, cardiovascular disease, diabetes, AIDS, violence, and infant mortality (Kritek et al., 2002). Twenty-five percent of black women over the age of 55 have diabetes; only 72% of black women with breast cancer compared to 87% of white women with breast cancer are likely to survive 5 years after diagnosis (AHRQ website). The mortality rate is higher for black women even though the actual incidence of breast cancer is lower than among white non-Hispanics (Miller, Kolonel, Bernstein, Young, Swanson, & West, 1996); and between 1987 and 1995, over 34% of non-Hispanic black women and 22% of Hispanic women had high blood pressure, compared to 19% of white women (Centers for Disease Control and Prevention).

Access to Health Care

Members of minority groups have less access than whites to a usual source of primary health care. This helps explain the differences in mortality rates noted above. Non-Hispanic whites aged 50 to 64 are more likely to see a physician in an office setting than are Hispanics and African Americans of the same age. These latter groups are more likely to use clinics or hospital emergency rooms as their source of health care. Less than 16% of the white population relies on clinics or hospitals for health care, whereas 20% of African Americans and 30% of Hispanics do so (AARP, 2002; AHRQ website).

Quality of Care

Differences also exist in treatment received, which may also help account for disparity in survival rates. For instance, the length of time between abnormal mammography screening and follow-up testing to determine diagnosis of breast cancer is twice as long for Asian Americans, African Americans, and Hispanic women than it is for white women. African Americans with HIV infection are less likely to be on antiretroviral therapy and less likely to be receiving protease inhibitors than others with HIV (AHRQ website), whereas African Americans with heart disease are 13% less likely to undergo coronary angioplasty and one-third less likely to undergo bypass surgery than whites with heart disease. Among African Americans, women are less likely than other women and men of all groups to have access to life-saving therapies for heart attacks (Canto et al., 2000).

Meanwhile, a recent study in Boston, funded by the AHRQ, found that African-American hospital patients receive a lower quality of care than their white counterparts. Disparities continue to exist even within nursing facilities. Asian Americans, Hispanic, and African-American nursing home residents are far less likely than white residents to have sensory and communication aids such as glasses and hearing aids (AHRQ website).

Causes of Disparities

Medicare is an almost universal health insurance program for those over 65, but significant differences persist in this age group in health status, access to care, and outcomes among minority populations (Institute for Medicare Practice, 1999). Causes of these disparities are varied and include lack of financial resources, uneven access to health insurance, discrimination, and cultural and communication barriers.

Financial Resources

Minority populations are overrepresented among the poor and lowest income groups in the U.S. In a society in which even health insurance does not guarantee full coverage of medical/health costs and copayments are rising along with overall health costs, it is not surprising that many choose not to seek medical assistance except in emergency circumstances. How much the lack of preventive care contributes to poor health in old age is difficult to measure accurately but few doubt that poor health and lack of early detection of disease are linked to low financial resources.

Health Insurance

In spite of Medicare for those over 65 years of age and Medicaid coverage for various special populations and many children, a full 15% of the U.S. population is without health insurance. The percentages are even higher among minority groups. Dr. Mohammad Akhter, immediate past Executive Director of the American Public Health Association, notes that one fifth (20%) of African Americans and one third (33%) of Latinos have no health insurance (Bashir, 2002). Black women are twice as likely and Hispanic women three times as likely to be uninsured compared to white women.

Furthermore, health insurance coverage has declined in the past two years. Those with health insurance are increasingly discovering that their employer-based plan no longer covers as much of the health care costs as formerly, and many who once had coverage now no longer do so. A full 37% of Hispanic men have no coverage today (AHRQ website). This is due to the rise in unemployment and loss of persons from the labor market and their accompanying health insurance, as well as to the economic decline,which translates into lower incomes with which to purchase health insurance. Additionally, minority persons are more likely than whites to leave the labor force and their health insurance coverage via the involuntary pathway of existing poor health (Flippen & Tienda, 2002). The result is even poorer health. Health insurance contributes independently to better health. "The uninsured receive too little care, too late. They receive poorer quality care; they are sicker and die sooner" (Kotelchuck, 2003).

Discrimination and Cultural and Communication Barriers

Discrimination, whether it is institutional or individual, is frequently a barrier that may hinder minority persons from seeking health care and/ or lead to a lower level of care from health care professionals and institutions. At the institutional level, the values, research interests, and even funding sources may not be cognizant of or interested in meeting the health needs of minority groups. Members of minority groups are unlikely to believe that the institution is welcoming or even relevant to their health concerns. Equally common are individual cultural and communication barriers. Language differences can prove insurmountable. If staff at hospitals, clinics, and medical practices cannot communicate in the native language(s) of their patients, health care is compromised. Communication goes beyond being able to understand one another in a common language to include understanding of the mores and beliefs of other cultures. Health beliefs, expectations, and assumptions are all culturally based and there can be divergent views of what constitutes "healthy." These differences need to be recognized, acknowledged, and respected to enable appropriate health assessment, diagnosis, care, and patient compliance with the treatment regimen.

Solutions

In the spring of 2001, the National Center for Minority Health and Health Disparities (NIH) funded a series of national conferences, each focused on a specific population. Two hundred and fifty persons attended the conference focused on women of color. Its central themes were "access issues and cultural incompetence as deterrents to the elimination of health disparities and on education, funding, and community-based, community-driven research as mechanisms for change" (Kritek et al., 2002). Recommended strategies to overcome the disparities in health include expanding the role of minority communities in the planning and delivery of care, changing health care itself, and changing how things get done. The conclusions the conference participants reached and their recommendations for change are equally valid for all minority populations, as the conveners themselves suggested. "The health care disparities among women of color are for us simply one aspect of the larger issue of health care disparities among people of color" (Kritek et al.).

Improving Access

On the societal level, legislating health insurance coverage for all, regardless of employment status or income, and rectifying the inequality in allocation of resources to ensure that the latest technology and advances are readily available in all communities, will go a long way to overcoming the current health disparities. Perhaps more important are changes at the local level that foster health care that relates to the patients' values and culture. Health care environments that are gender and culture sensitive need to be created. This can be accomplished by increasing the number of health care providers from minority populations, training non-minority health care providers in cultural competence, employing community members from within the patient population as case managers and receptionists, and using the language(s) of the local community on forms, public signs, and in outreach/publicity materials.

Heath care provided in a community by community members is perhaps the most effective means of encouraging utilization of health care services by members of minority populations. Studies have shown the value of the delivery of mammograms for minority women at the community level, sometimes using mobile trailers and rooms in neighborhood centers and religious organizations (Siegel & Clancy, 2002). Health fairs, which offer health screening, consultation, and information within the local community, are very well attended. Health care systems are advised to partner with social services at the neighborhood level in order to accomplish a community-based modality. "Co-ordina-

tion between health and social service networks may be vital to enhancing health in our most vulnerable populations" (Buelow, Zimmer,
Mellor, & Sax, 1998).

Improving Cultural Competence

Education is a major strategy in reducing adverse stereotyping between
cultures and increasing understanding. This education goes beyond
mere learning of facts about others' cultural beliefs and mores to an in-
depth understanding of the role of culture in the lives of all individuals.
Understanding the role of one's own culture in forming oneself is the
key to a beginning appreciation and comprehension of others. Because
health beliefs and concepts are culturally driven, it behooves all health
care and social service providers to become culturally competent.

Improving Healthy Behaviors

Many of the health conditions in which disparities exist between minorities and whites can be improved by individual changes in behaviors and
practices. Equally true for whites, good nutrition, exercise, avoidance
of smoking, and reduction of stress can lower the incidence of conditions such as diabetes and heart disease. The AARP National Research
Center on Health Promotion and Aging strongly advises promotion of
these practices and behaviors via health promotion programs that take
into consideration the characteristics of their targeted groups. The
Center notes that ethnic groups are diverse and so any health promotion
campaigns must also be diverse in method and form of outreach and
implementation. Once more, solutions lead back to the community, at
which level the most appropriate and relevant outreach for the local
minority population can be initiated.

Improving the Environment

There is growing realization of and popular media attention to the
impact of environment on health and unhealthy behaviors. Obesity,
asthma, diabetes, and heart disease are increasingly prevalent, and many
believe this increase in incidence is due to the manner in which our
environments are designed (New York Academy of Medicine, 2003).
Where there are no sidewalks or bike paths and in sprawling communities where stores are clustered in shopping malls, there is universal

reliance on driving, which means less walking exercise and more air pollution. It may be no coincidence that those living in rural areas without easy transportation or in cities that accommodate walking over the automobile, tend to live longer than the average American. Environmental design impacts the health of all ethnic groups but, whether due to low income, recent immigration, or housing racism, minority groups frequently live in crowded inner city areas, subject to old housing stock and pollution. Changes in environmental design may be part of the solution to eliminating health disparities among all populations.

Conclusion

The conference on eliminating health disparities among minority women recommended making health care more "family focused, more patient friendly, more community-based, and more cognizant of a woman's right to choose" (Kritek et al., 2002)—almost exactly the same principles underscored by the Baby Boomers attending the Summit meetings on which this publication is based.

The conference conveners concluded their report on the conference deliberations as follows:

> The biggest issue we face in resolving this issue (eliminating health disparities among minority women) is the cultural insensitivity and incompetence of existing educational and health care delivery structures. Their values, funding patterns, research, care programs, and underlying discriminatory practices are our main deterrent in accessing the care we seek. We want to eliminate health disparities for people of color, and we recognize that we will need educational programs, funding, and programs of research to do this. We would actually prefer to promote health and prevent disease. We know most of all that we need to do it on our terms, in our communities, under our leadership and control. [Kritek et al., 2002]

TODAY'S OLDER POPULATION

At the time of the 2000 census, almost 13% of the U.S. population was over 65 years of age—35 million persons. With today's life expectancy now at 83 years, those reaching 65 years of age can anticipate 18 more years of life on average. Racially, ethnically, and economically diverse, the older population spans two to three generations of persons from

65 to over 100 years old. There are already over 68,000 U.S. centenarians and the number continues to grow. Five to six percent of all older persons receive institutional care at any one period of time and of the remaining 84–85% living in the community, one third live alone, two thirds with others—spouse, other family members or friends.

Although the majority of today's elderly are not at risk financially, 12% are at or below the poverty line and a full one third of all those over 75 years of age are considered poor. The rate of poverty increases with each decade of life with women, earning less and living longer than men, the most vulnerable.

This current group of older persons are the first to experience the advances in medicine, technology, and public health that have extended the life expectancy, enabling many who might have died in the past at earlier ages of heart disease, stroke, or age-related diseases to continue living into their late eighties and beyond, while managing chronic diseases. Over two thirds of the current older population state that their health is good, very good, or excellent, in spite of the fact that most older people suffer from at least one chronic health condition and one third, mostly among the ranks of the over-85-year-olds, say that they are handicapped in some way from one or more chronic conditions, such as hypertension, heart disease, or arthritis.

Not unexpectedly, older persons with low income are less healthy and suffer more chronic illnesses than their peers. Also troubling is the well-documented racial and ethnic disparity in access, availability, and quality of health care. Even when care is available, health care providers are not educationally prepared for the various cultural and ethnic populations that they treat, perhaps thereby contributing to the disparity in quality of care.

In spite of older persons frequently living many years with chronic illness, the current U.S. health care system is focused on acute care. Chronic illness and social or functional limitations are not widely addressed. Our health care system still remains fragmented, and comprehensive health care, recognized as the optimum mode for delivery of care to older persons, is rarely actualized. Where it does exist, it is at risk, being eroded by increasing health costs and the competing interests of the managed care organizations and health insurance companies.

Currently, Medicare recipients spend 50% of their income out of pocket for health care. Medicare coverage has failed to keep pace with increasing health care costs so that there is only partial coverage for most care. As a result, growing numbers of physicians and HMOs are dropping Medicare patients or are refusing to take them. There is a movement, at the national policy level, toward privatization. For example, the Federal administration has proposed linking coverage of prescription drugs to registration in Health Maintenance Organizations (HMOs) but it is not at all clear whether Medicare recipients will be able to find HMOs interested in accepting them. In the past few years, a number of HMOs have turned away from insuring older persons as being too costly and a drain on resources.

Utilization of nursing homes has decreased over the last ten years, reflecting a drop in disability rates among the older population. This reduced nursing home utilization has occurred without a corresponding increase in the supply of community-based health services, although Medicare is covering more home care than in the past. For those frail elderly requiring nursing home care, the level of care is deemed inadequate. The recent Federal Report on Nursing Home Staffing found inadequate staffing in 90% of the approximately 17,000 nursing homes in the U.S. that together serve 1.5 million residents. The report concludes that understaffing places residents at significant risk for health problems such as "bedsores, bloodborne infections, dehydration, malnutrition, and pneumonia" (Fleck, 2003).

Baby Boomers as Our Future Older Population

Based on actuarial calculations of the current 76 million Baby Boomers, 69–70 million will survive to age 65. Projected life expectancy by the time Baby Boomers reach old age is 84 for women and 78 for men. Baby Boomers will enter the ranks of older persons in 2011 and continue to increase the numbers of U.S. elderly until 2030, contributing to the estimate that by 2020, there will be 7 to 9 million persons over the age of 85 years, and twenty years later, by 2050, 835,000 persons over the age of 100.

In the main, these older persons will prove themselves healthier, better educated, more active, and more productive than their grandparents and parents. As a group, however, they will exhibit wide differences and even greater racial, ethnic, cultural, and economic diversity and health status.

Health

The majority of these aging Baby Boomers will do well through their seventies. However, by 2020, it is anticipated that 50% of the 7–9 million people over 85 will need some level of help. Though they are healthier than our current older population, chronic illnesses will remain prevalent, especially or perhaps because older persons will be living longer and will therefore be at greater risk. Today the majority of those over 50 are living with at least one chronic health condition. Only 30% of the 50–64 age group (the leading edge of the Baby Boomers) is free of chronic conditions, disabilities, and functional limitations (AARP, 2002), meaning that the majority will reach old age with existing functional limitations and health concerns.

Diseases and disabilities expected to occur among the Baby Boomers as older persons include malignant neoplasms, coronary diseases, cerebrovascular disorders, orthopedic/arthritic impairments, cognitive impairment disorders (14 million persons are projected to be suffering from Alzheimer's disease by 2040), visual and auditory disorders, and depression, with over 9 million older persons with mental illness (Shea, 2003). These are all conditions that can impact Activities of Daily Living (ADLs) and create a need for caregiving assistance, whether from the informal system of family and friends or from the formal system of paid care providers.

Today's escalating costs threaten drug needs and access and quality of care, and it is predicted that this trend will continue. Though needed, there is little current promise that future health care insurance will cover "continuity of care," the support provided by caregivers, adult day health care, or health education. In spite of the national debate, few have expectations that prescription drugs will be fully covered. Projections indicate that by 2025, elderly Medicare beneficiaries will be spending 30% of their income on health care (AARP, 2002).

The large Baby Boom generation contributed to a second peak in births when it entered its child-bearing years. Overall, however, there has been a drop in fertility rates, which portends both shortages in the U.S. health care labor force and fewer family members to provide informal, unpaid care. There is already a shortage of nurses, which is expected to become even more acute as we move through this decade. Furthermore, the current U.S. policy of controlled immigration may keep replacements in short supply. Baby Boomers themselves are already spending a greater length of time than the preceding generation as part of the "sandwich" cohort, caring for both children and elderly parents. These Baby Boomers sometimes worry over who will be available to provide care for them when they reach their eighties.

Income

It is expected that there will be increasing income disparity between the economically secure and those in poverty. Looking at the economic status of Baby Boomers, it appears that the top one fifth will have a secure future, with financial independence in retirement. In contrast, the lowest one fourth will face a difficult future, dependent on continuing work opportunities and public retirement and low income programs (i.e., Social Security, SSI and Medicaid) (AARP, 1999). Women, in particular, will face economic problems and fall into poverty. Today's job mobility and high unemployment rate suggest uncertainty about future income available for retirement from Social Security, pensions, and savings. At the same time, health costs are expected to increase, while the current trend of decreased coverage by employers is also expected to continue into the foreseeable future.

Work/Retirement

Women will continue in the labor market, many working beyond 65 years of age, perhaps more for financial reasons than the desire to continue working as an end in itself. The tendency to frequent job changes for both men and women will continue, perhaps becoming even more common. Many can expect 5 to 6 job changes during their working years.

Unlike popular belief, recent surveys suggest that many of today's Baby Boomers will be somewhat prepared for their transition into retirement. Baby Boomers are thinking ahead in terms of income and, if financially able, are saving to ensure sufficient income for their non-working years. There is uncertainty about the status of Social Security. Those who believe they will have insufficient funds are concerned, and their plans for the retirement years frequently include part-time work or self-employment. Planning ahead for other aspects of retirement is less common. Baby Boomers, on the whole, are ill-prepared, emotionally and physically, for retirement and are giving little consideration to potential future health needs and costs (AARP, 1999).

Housing and Lifestyles

Living conditions for Baby Boomers will be better than they are for today's older population. A full 60% will be living independently but alone, which may well presage increased social isolation. Baby Boomers have raised fewer children than their parents and this, coupled with the intergenerational distancing due to increased mobility, indicates that members of an extended family may be unavailable to provide assistance and care when it is needed.

On the other hand, longevity itself and our changing concept of the family may offset the negative impact of children at a distance. Older persons of the future are likely to find themselves members of four and five generation families, encompassing many adult family members. The entire notion of the nuclear family has altered due to the frequency of divorce, same-gender cohabitation, remarriages, and step-family con-figurations. In spite of bearing fewer children, Baby Boomers may lay claim to many close familial contacts. The growth in single parenthood also suggests that Baby Boomers will participate in grandparenting and great-grandparenting roles to a greater degree than their own par-ents did.

SUMMARY

The current older U.S. population is living longer than ever before and the trend is expected to continue, with the Baby Boomers experiencing an even longer life expectancy. If the Baby Boomers are unprepared for old age, it is also true that today's society is unprepared for this longevity revolution. Very few individuals, governmental bodies, busi-nesses, or non-profit institutions are seriously dealing with the universal challenge of longevity, population aging, and the myriad questions that must be answered. For example only 2% of all foundation money in this country goes to the field of aging. A kind of society-wide denial is operative that confounds the imagination and cruelly leaves our future older population vulnerable to whatever vicissitudes may lie ahead (But-ler, 2001).

On the individual, personal level, we have insufficient role models or even a generally accepted understanding of what it may mean to live into our eighties and our nineties. The U.S. remains an ageist society, viewing older persons as irrelevant or, when productive and creative into their older years, as amazing phenomena. There are signs that this is changing, and dim shadows are coming into focus to provide us with a more realistic view. Though the Baby Boomers themselves share in these ageist attitudes, it is their initiation into old age that promises to be the strongest force to change society's perspective and "tell it like it is."

REFERENCES

AARP. (1999). *Boomers approaching midlife: How secure a future?* Public Policy Institute. Washington, DC: AARP's Public Policy Institute.

AARP. (2001). *In the middle: A report on multicultural boomers coping with family and aging issues. National survey.* Washington, DC: Author.

AARP. (2002). *Beyond 50:02: A report to the nation on trends in health security.* Washington, DC: Author.

Agency for Healthcare Research and Quality (AHRQ) website. (2003). Retrieved September 15, 2003, from www.ahrq.gov/research/disparit.htm

Bashir, S. (2002). Principled professionalism: The American face of public health, Dr. Mohammad Akhter. *American Journal of Public Health, 92*(12), 1012.

Buelow, J., Zimmer, A., Mellor, M. J., & Sax, R. (1998). Mammography screening for older minority women. *Journal of Applied Gerontology, 17*(2), 133–149.

Butler, R. N. (2001, October 10). *Seven deadly issues.* Keynote address at summit meeting: *Can my eighties be like my fifties?* The New York Academy of Medicine, New York, NY.

Canto, J., Allison, J., Kiefe, C., Fincher, C., Farmer, R., Sekar, P., et al. (2000). *New England Journal of Medicine, 342*(15), 1094–1100.

Centers for Disease Control and Prevention, Department of Health and Human Services. http://www.cdc.gov

Crimmins, E. M., & Saito, Y. (2001). Trends in healthy life expectancy in the United States, 1970–1990: Gender, racial, and educational differences. *Social Science and Medicine, 52,* 1629–1641.

Cutler, N. E. (1998, Spring). Preparing for their older years: The financial diversity of aging boomers. *Generations: Journal of the American Society on Aging, 22*(1), 1–86.

Fleck, C. (2003, June 6). Your health. Nursing home care is found wanting. *AARP Bulletin Online.* Retrieved November 21, 2003, from http://www.aarp.org/bulletin/yourhealth/Articles/a2003-06-23-nursinghome.html

Flippen, C., & Tienda, M. (2002). Raising retirement age weakens safety net for workers of color and pathways to retirement. *Public Policy and Aging Report,* National Academy of an Aging Society, Gerontological Society of America.

Institute for Medicare Practice. (1999). *Health care disparities among Medicare beneficiaries: Overcoming barriers of race, ethnicity and socioeconomic status.* Institute for Medicare Practice, Mount Sinai School of Medicine, New York, NY, November 9.

Koop, E. (2003). website http://www.drkoop.com

Kotelchuck, R. (2003). *The consequences of uninsurance: A shared destiny.* Report by the Institute of Medicine Subcommittee on the Community, Institute of Medicine of the National Academies. Key Findings, Report #2. *Care without coverage: Too little, too late.* Slide 8. New York, NY. Presentation March 11.

Kritek, P., Hargraves, M., Cuellar, E., Dallo, F., Gauthier, D., Holland, C., et al. (2002). Eliminating health disparities among minority women: A report on conference workshop process and outcomes. *American Journal of Public Health, 92*(4), 580–587.

Miller, B. A., Kolonel, L. N., Bernstein, L., Young, J. L., Jr., Swanson, G. M., West, D., et al. (Eds.). (1996). *Racial/ethnic patterns of cancer in the United States, 1988–1992.* Bethesda, MD: National Cancer Institute (NIH Publication No. 96-4104).

New York Academy of Medicine Newsletter. (2003, summer). Experts explore links between health problems and the built environment. *Notes*, 3–4.

Shea, D. G. (2003). Swimming upstream: Geriatric mental health workforce. *Public Policy and Aging Report, 13*(2), 3–7. National Academy on an Aging Society.

Siegel, J., & Clancy, C. (2002). Community-based interventions: Taking on the cost and cost-effectiveness questions. *Health Service Research, 35*(5), 905–909. AHRQ Publication No. 01-R032. Washington, DC.

U.S. Census. (2000). See http://www.census.gov http://www.aoa.gov

U.S. Department of Health and Human Services. (1985). *Report of the Secretary's task force on black and minority health.* Rockville, MD.

Chapter 3

A Baby Boomer's Perception of the Baby Boom Era

Sue Woodman

I am a perfect example of the aging Baby Boomer. Born at the start of the 1950s, I was among the first generation to be given the luxury of preventive medicine in childhood, from polio shots to free milk in school. I came of age in the 1960s, and in my twenties, I took the Pill, had a few sexual partners, and smoked, both cigarettes and pot. In my thirties, I stopped smoking, got married, and had children. I was a proud practitioner of natural childbirth and breast-feeding. I started working out and taking vitamins. In my forties, I dealt with the care and death of ailing relatives. Now that I am entering my fifties, I am hitting menopause just as programmed. I have great triceps thanks to my health club membership, and more than a passing interest in plastic surgery. For all these reasons, I am a worthy representative of my generation.

The Baby Boomer generation—the 76 million strong cohort of babies born in the 20 years after World War II—has been much studied over the years. The sheer weight of our numbers has guaranteed that our every step along life's highway has marked a demographic trend: from how old we were when we had our babies to how young we want to be when we retire.

Over the past three decades, plenty has been documented and written about our generation. It is suggested that we are the most privileged and self-obsessed generation of all time, we elbow everyone else out of the way, we are indulged babies who continue to cling to faded images of a bygone youth culture. This may be because we grew up during one of those eras when the forces of history and geography came together. The zeitgeist in the '60s and early '70s was all about youth, and there we young people were, living in a society of postwar plenty, with infinite opportunity to explore our limits. Which we did. With sex, drugs, and a strong sense of entitlement. What we wanted—what we still want—was, simply, complete control over all aspects of our lives. And the tightest focus of our control has always been our health.

For most Boomers, health has meant politics. Remember the feminist mantra, "The Personal is Political," and our '70s refrain, "Our Bodies, Ourselves"? It began with sexual politics and expanded into all areas of our health care, as we have passed through each milestone of life. The sexual revolution, the abortion movement, the vast campaign for breast cancer funding, activism over AIDS research, and now, a fast-growing market in anti-aging medicine—all arising out of the patient-empowerment movement that began with feminist Baby Boomers. That movement challenged the medical establishment every step of the way, and, in so doing, has contributed to some of the most sweeping changes in modern health care.

Take the sexual revolution. It was fueled by the advent of the Pill, the most reliable contraceptive yet invented. What we did not know was that sexual promiscuity would lead to a bedful of new sexually transmitted diseases. At the start of the '60s, there were just two of them—gonorrhea and syphilis, both of which were treatable with anti-biotics. By the end of the '70s, there were nine strains of sexual infections, many of them incurable, such as herpes, and some even potentially deadly, such as the human papilloma virus, which can cause cancerous changes in cervical cells.

For most Boomers, the wild times seemed to end when we began having children. We were late coming to that, compared to other generations, but when we got there, we stormed the barricades. We revolutionized childbirth by making it natural again and refusing to lie down to do it. We wanted—and got—Lamaze classes, birthing rooms, midwives. We rejected the accepted wisdom about baby formulas and insisted on breast feeding—in New York, we even changed laws to allow us to do it in public. We challenged the medical profession over the need for Cesareans.

But it was not all positive. One immediate effect of our delayed childbearing was an apparent higher incidence of infertility, which, in turn, spawned a vastly lucrative science of conception. It's impossible to count the number of couples with infertility problems at any given time, but experts believe infertility became more widespread in the late '70s and early '80s—the very period in which Boomer women were having babies. The experts believe this was at least partly due to the ravages of those "new" sexually transmitted diseases.

But then, along came the science. The first test tube baby was born in 1978, and soon, thousands of American women wanted one too. Finally, science and the marketplace could combine to offer new hope for couples denied the baby of their dreams. Expensive clinics popped up coast to coast, with varying reputations: The doctors with the greatest number of smiling baby pictures in their waiting rooms were the rock stars of their profession, with desperate women pleading to receive treatment. Even approaching 50, Boomers continue to make demands on the baby doctors. Not prepared to take no for an answer, many Boomers are pushing the limits of childbearing well into another decade. In 2000, more than 3,000 women aged 50 or above had babies. No statistics were kept prior to this because postmenopausal motherhood was just too rare. Fertility experts have worked hard to make everything possible. They are currently working on ways to inject the DNA from a prospective mother into the eggs of a surrogate donor so that her baby will be genetically her own.

Another part of the sociological puzzle that marked the Boomers as a particular generation was drugs. We were the generation that took drugs in fistfuls, and we paid a high price in overdoses and ruined lives. But it is also arguable that Boomers' experiences with drugs have resulted in social good as well as harm. Most notably, our excesses have resulted in a sophisticated science of drug addiction with a profoundly more compassionate understanding of addiction's nature and causes than ever before.

Today's breakthroughs in brain imaging technology enable us to better understand exactly what drugs can do to our brain cells. The 4,000-plus existing studies on marijuana make it among the most studied substances in medicine, and there is now a flurry of new research underway on the effects, both therapeutic and harmful, of various illegal drugs. Epidemiological proof rests with the generation who actually tried them—Boomers. We are the human guinea pigs, and the years ahead will answer the question: How have recreational drugs made us the worse for wear?

There's plenty of evidence that Boomers are still turning to drugs, albeit different ones these days. More middle-aged people are now taking antidepressants than ever before. That may be because drugs such as Prozac and Paxil have fewer side effects and are easier to tolerate than antidepression medications of the past. It may also be that Boomers want and expect to feel better. Are we not entitled to this? The use of these new generation antidepressants has begun a fascinating dialogue about humankind's right to pursue happiness as an integral part of good health. Which is also what psychotherapy, the holistic health movement, and tummy tucks are all about.

Of course, all these things are also about middle age. The Boomers are discovering that for those who did not die before they got old, the struggle to hold on to our youth is presenting us with new health challenges.

The first one is to "make over" menopause, just as we did the earlier milestones. This means taking on the complex, urgent topic of hormone replacement therapy. The estrogen replacement drug, Premarin, is the most heavily prescribed drug in America, with over 10 million U.S. women taking it every day even though the vast majority of women who start taking it stop doing so because they are uncomfortable with the various side effects.

New evidence shows that estrogen's side effects may outweigh its benefits, and that it may be more dangerous to take it than not to. For years, physicians and their patients accepted the finding that estrogen protected women's hearts after menopause. Now repeated studies are showing us that it does not. What the millions of Boomer women approaching menopause need now is to be given clearer recommendations, based on today's better understanding of what hormonal replacement involves.

Middle-aged men are luckier than women. First, we know more about managing their health—their hearts, their drug reactions, and their pain thresholds—because most research has focused on them. Second, they have been blessed with a little blue diamond-shaped pill called Viagra. Viagra was discovered by accident in 1998, and has quickly become a pharmaceutical blockbuster with an estimated 10 million prescriptions filled every year. The real phenomenon of Viagra was that no one guessed so many men would want it, but as soon as a remedy became available, men came forward to get it. Now, the pharmaceutical companies are confident that a magic bullet for women—a little pink heart-shaped pill, perhaps—will be another, maybe even bigger, goldmine. So far, the female version of love potion number nine has proved elusive. But in the past three years, sexual health clinics have sprung up from coast to coast to try to analyze the physical ingredients of desire in menopausal women and to replace those that have diminished. This has led in turn to a fascinating debate about what is normal, and what we "medicalize" and then seek to cure. It has also led the experts into discussing the components of female sexuality: physical versus emotional. Yet another new avenue for science to map in coming years.

We are lucky to find ourselves, once again, in one of those symbiotic eras when scientific understanding is exploding right alongside demand. Genetic decoding, surgical and pharmaceutical innovations, and the fast-growing understanding of the brain are all taking off just as boomers are entering the disease stage, becoming depressed, and demanding results. Over the past decade, the field of anti-aging medicine has made dramatic leaps. It's still an unproven science, but we are all believers. We have been willing to try anything, alternative remedies such as acupuncture and homeopathy, herbal supplements (which now generate around $600 million annually), and a vast fitness industry that we are relying on to help us age less catastrophically than our parents' generation.

Thanks to Jane Fonda and the long line of fitness gurus who followed her in the early '80s, most Boomers have grown up in a culture of "Use it or Lose it," and according to the International Health, Racquet and Sports Club Association, Boomers make up the largest percentage of health club members in the country, and their numbers have grown 107% over the past decade. We know that lifting weights guards against osteoporosis, and that moderate exercise raises metabolism, good cholesterol, and mood. Unfortunately, prolonged years of high-impact exercise have also worn out our knees and ankles at a record rate. Doctors are now advising their middle-aged patients to switch from running and basketball to more joint-friendly activities like cycling, to avoid the condition with the eloquent name—Boomeritis. But even in this area, there have been developments to help us. Arthroscopic surgery has made huge progress in terms of its minimally invasive techniques and what it can do to help and, not surprisingly, we Boomers are the largest group to take advantage of this progress.

The growth of the fitness movement poses a central quandary about Boomers. On the one hand, we are health obsessed and turning to soy and yoga as never before. On the other hand, the nation as a whole is becoming more sedentary, more overweight, and consequently more prone to heart disease and diabetes. The U.S. now leads the way in what the World Health Organization proclaims is a worldwide epidemic of obesity.

Some of the fault may rest with the way the media cover health. Health reporting has become a huge journalistic field over the past couple of decades, in both print and broadcasting, from philosophical considerations of medicine in the *New Yorker* to bunion advice on your local newscast. But I believe that the way health tends to get covered often misrepresents the big picture. We are given daily promises about breakthroughs based on single studies of sometimes fewer than a couple of dozens patients. We are given a lot of meaningless information dressed up as science. I recently saw a report on a study that showed that eating with low lights causes some people to binge, whereas eating in bright light helps them eat less. Other studies state that the nation is in a state of chronic fatigue; yet people who sleep more than eight hours a night die earlier. What are we to do? Remain fatigued or die earlier? Can eating under bright lights really make a serious difference to our weight problems, or is it just a distraction from the unpleasant, indisputable truth about eating—which is that if we need to eat less, we have to do just that? As Americans and Boomers, we would rather rely on science to find alternatives, such as fat-free banana sundaes and meatless chicken breasts, rather than simply do without.

The wealth of reporting confuses, and promises more than can actually be delivered. We believe that science has an answer for everything or will have within the next five years and all we need to do is just to keep going until then. The reporting obscures the forest for the trees. Why do the magazines that purport to give us health information still carry cigarette ads? And why do we continue to let the media dictate a powerful, subliminal ageism message that to be old is to be worthless, but that luckily, there are products on hand to help?

One of the most interesting aspects of the health media is their celebrities: Andrew Weill, with his holistic beliefs, and his extensive study of psychedelic drugs; Deepak Chopra, who has combined successful Western self-promotion techniques with Eastern philosophical tenets on health and anti-aging; Christiane Northrup, part careerist, part earth-mother, with her integrative mind/body approach to women's health; and the immeasurably influential Oprah Winfrey, whose show has made all these practitioners the health superstars they are. What is the secret of their success? Maybe it's the irresistible message they all share that aging may be largely a state of mind, and, consequently, within our control. Handle stress better, eat better, exercise, and breathe deeply and you may stay forever young.

No generation has been so eager to buy into that belief as we are. Plastic surgery, Dead Sea rejuvenating skin wraps, hair regrowth products, Viagra. The fact is that we really do not want to get older, let alone old. So we experience it, kicking and screaming, refusing to go quietly into that good night, just as we have refused to go everywhere else. But if we can pull it off, if we can really bring about some changes in the transition to old age, then this final act of rebellion may turn out to be our most important legacy. The Youth Generation: who would have thought it?

As we watch our parents reach the end of their lives, many of us are scared of their physical decrepitude—their cardiovascular disease, their osteoporosis, and all the accumulated deficits of those so-called golden years. For me, the hardest thing to witness is the isolation and loneliness that seem to accompany old age. Independence is the preferred goal but for many old people today, the advantages of remaining independent are overwhelmed by the difficulties of being alone. At a time of rising health care costs, many elderly people are further isolated because they cannot afford the help they need. Maybe, we say to our friends, our old age will be the time to live communally. And maybe the culture of therapy and confession, that we and Oprah have espoused, will help us to reach out for support and company as our mobility declines.

The public health organizations, responsible for preparing the nation for the huge generation of elderly that we will become, are hoping that will take a long time. They are planning to redesign communities to encourage movement, to improve access to wellness centers and footpaths, and to keep us as sprightly as possible for as long as possible. There are already many retirement communities around the country that have transformed the image of old age homes into Club Med holiday resorts, offering sports facilities, social events, and, above all, the daily companionship of others. The mental health component of aging is so important and still so overlooked. I hope that our growing understanding of the aging body and brain is in time to help us cope with the existential miseries of being old, as well as the physical ones. (This wish, in itself, immediately identifies me as a typical Boomer.)

After old age, death. When the end comes, it will not be surprising to find us Boomers demanding control over our deaths, just as we have over every stage of our lives. It's already happening, largely thanks to Boomer-aged doctors like Joanne Lynn in Washington, Diane Meier in

New York, and numerous others around the U.S. who are changing their profession's approach to end-of-life care and removing the cultural taboo surrounding death. To modern medicine, death is an invincible foe, for science just cannot beat it, and always suffers defeat. Now, medical students are being taught how to accept and discuss it. Hospice care is becoming more popular among terminally ill patients, and more health care providers are accepting their valuable role. Patients can draw up end-of-life directives, and doctors who fail to heed them can be prosecuted. Over the past few years, laws have been passed in Oregon and in several European countries allowing doctors to prescribe lethal drugs to people already in the final stages of illness.

The Right to Die movement has been fueled by the development of sophisticated medical technology that enables doctors to prolong life as never before. But there are many people (surveys suggest the majority of Americans) who prefer not to have their lives sustained by machines, and who are determined not to allow this to happen to themselves. That's why activists are working on creating a "suicide pill," a lethal substance, or combination of substances, that people can obtain without a prescription, to enable them to take their own actions to end their lives. In fact, a range of products are being developed such as plastic bags with Velcro fastenings, adaptations of scuba diving masks, and high-altitude tents that gradually remove oxygen from the air supply for people to use when they wish to die. This is taking our buying power to its literal limit. We can even become consumers of death.

With the Boomers' history of activism in all areas of health care, this growing involvement with the manner of our deaths seems an inevitable final chapter. But I am putting my money on the pharmaceutical industry bailing us out at the last minute. The genetically engineered, three-a-day-for-maximum-effect Eternal Life capsules they will be producing any day now will be expensive, of course, but we Boomers will have our credit cards ready.

Chapter 4

Income Security: Social Security, Work, Pensions, and Savings

> Social Security, Medicare, Medicaid—I believe they are the three cylinders that fuel the American dream. . . . We must not allow our rendezvous with destiny to become a rendezvous with poverty and disease again.
>
> Donna Shalala

> The crisis in Social Security and Medicare is a political, not an economic, phenomenon.
>
> Bruce Vladeck

At the beginning of the twenty-first century, we can look back at the preceding one as an era of major advances in government's responsibility for social welfare. It was a time in which the United States "transformed the experience of growing old. We ended the bread lines and the poor houses. We replaced dependence with independence. We made healthcare a right for our seniors and the disabled. We established retirement as an expected part of the lifecycle. These are in fact historic achievements. They define the last century and define us as Americans" (Shalala, 2002). Social Security, Medicare, Med-

icaid, and availability of health insurance are all aspects of industrialized America that today we view as rights. And yet, at the dawn of
the new century, we are concerned about the continuing viability of
many of these programs and express growing uncertainty about their
future. Baby Boomers worry whether these programs will be there for
them when they become old and, if they are, whether they will be adequate.

Today's Baby Boomers number 76 million. By the time they reach
65 years of age, this number will have dropped to approximately 69 to
70 million as the inevitability of illness and death takes its toll. Even
with this drop, the number of older persons in our future will be twice
as many as today. Economic and health circumstances change little for
the majority of persons when they reach 65 years of age, but as we
become older and enter our eighties, we can anticipate growing economic stress and declining health. Boomers born in 1946, at the beginning of the Baby Boom, will reach 80 years of age in 2026, a quarter
of a century in the future when we can expect society to be very different
than it is now. The youngest of the Boomers, born in 1964, will reach
80 years of age in 2044, almost mid-century. By this time, the U.S.
population will be extraordinarily diverse, and those people we today
call minorities will in fact number close to the majority of the population.
Mid-century will be vastly different from today in this respect and in
many more ways of which we cannot yet conceive. How will our older
population fare?

Whereas Baby Boomers may worry about the availability of Social
Security and Medicare when they reach retirement, others suggest that
it is the very existence of the Baby Boom generation itself, combined
with the increase in longevity, that will be responsible for any future
collapse of the programs. The sheer numbers of the generation threaten
to defeat the progress that was made in the last century toward individual
financial security in old age. The twentieth century began a process of
"mass-producing" older persons as a result of improved education, public health, and nutrition, as well as medical advances that have saved
the lives of mothers, the newborn, and, in the last half century, older
persons. Many diseases once defined as natural and inevitable have
proven preventable or treatable, and the life span of our ancestors,
threescore and ten, has been surpassed. This phenomenon is not unique
to the U.S. Soon the old will outnumber the young throughout the
industrialized world (Butler, 2001).

SOCIAL SECURITY AND PENSIONS

> Our overwhelming insistence on choosing old age over the alternative.
>
> Bruce Vladeck

Though Social Security remains strong today there is uncertainty about its ability to meet its fiscal responsibilities at the current level in the long run. Initiated in 1935, Social Security is a program the majority of Americans rely upon to help secure their financial security in retirement, and to be available as survivor benefits or in times of disability. Its existence effectively insures against poverty caused by retirement, death, or poor health. Financed by compulsory taxes on wages, Social Security is viewed as a right, and although the retirement benefits are no longer sufficient to secure financial security after retirement without the supplement of pensions and savings, few could manage financially without it. It is the largest single source of income for the elderly. It provides 38% of all income received by Americans over 65 years of age and nearly two thirds of SS beneficiaries receive more than half their income in Social Security payments (Purcell, 2001/2002). Without such payments, it is estimated that nearly half of all older Americans would be reduced to poverty.

IMPACT OF BABY BOOMERS ON SOCIAL SECURITY: DOOMSDAY OR ECONOMIC BLIP?

There is plenty of rhetoric on how Baby Boomers will cause a series of crises for our entitlement programs by the year 2030 because of "our overwhelming insistence on choosing old age over the alternative" (Vladeck, 2001). By 2032, the Baby Boomers, double the number of today's aged, will all have gained eligibility for Social Security under the prevailing regulations. The size of Social Security, therefore, is also likely to double. These projections have led "policy analysts, pundits and writers for the major newspaper editorial pages to identify the aging of the Baby Boomers as an enormous financial crisis . . . a source of various dire consequences" (Vladeck). This environment of doom has become the context within which to define the Baby Boomers.

Bruce Vladeck, former Director of the Health Care Financing Administration (HCFA) suggests several alternative, possibly more realistic, ways in which to think about and address the issues of aging Boomers. Vladeck reframes the issues, taking into consideration overlooked aspects that change the anticipated impact of the aging Baby Boomers on society and mitigate against future economic disaster.

The Cohort Phenomenon

The Baby Boomers are a cohort phenomenon, not a dramatic or permanent shift in the nature of life and the nature of democracy. Baby Boomers are not only substantially more numerous than any preceding generation but also substantially more numerous than any following generation. They had fewer children than their parents did. Beginning in the 1960s, just as the first wave of Baby Boomers reached childbearing age, there was a marked increase in the number of women not having any children (AARP, 2002), resulting in considerably smaller subsequent generations. Thus it can safely be predicted that the increased percentage of older persons in society, which we will witness from 2011 through 2030, will be a deviation from general population trends. The proportion of older persons to the rest of the U.S. population will increase, then level off and "become largely stable for the balance of the millennium, unless there is some additional major change in childbearing behavior, or in life expectancy, or in immigration policy" (Vladeck, 2001).

The cohort phenomenon has been apparent at every stage in the lives of the Baby Boomers. Predictions of what will happen with services and programs for the older population in the future are just more variants on what Baby Boomers have encountered throughout their lives. They were the first generation to go to elementary and secondary school routinely on double shifts, were responsible for a massive wave of school construction, competed for admission to college, entered the work force, and proceeded to hold down wages for all and to raise housing prices due to the sheer competition of numbers. Thus the anticipated pressure on Social Security can be viewed as a temporary cohort phenomenon that certainly requires forethought in planning but will not create a permanently catastrophic situation.

Aging Populations

The United States is not alone in the aging of its population. Japan, Sweden, and Western Germany are already close to experiencing 20%

of their populations over 65 years of age and by the end of another decade, nearly all the western European countries will have reached the twenty percentage mark. Japan, Sweden, and Western Germany appear to be managing without mass starvation, reactionary voting patterns, or other catastrophes. It is true that these countries differ from the U.S. in the ways they choose to provide income security and health care to their elderly but these differences are based on cultural, political, and economic variations rather than the fact that they are societies with almost one fifth of their populations defined as old.

Financial Predictions

The same forecasts that predict dire consequences as a result of a one hundred percent increase in the number of persons eligible for Social Security also suggest that "people of working age in 2030 and thereafter are going to be unimaginably rich by our current standards, at least on average" (Vladeck, 2001). The same models that show Social Security cash outlays doubling as a percent of Gross Domestic Product over the next forty years also show that real current dollar per capita income in the United States will increase between 50 and 100% over the same period of time. This means that the average household will have 50% to 100% more income to spend. By 2030, the United States will be at least twice as rich, per capita, as it is today, and the average household will have substantially more income. This has implications for the country's ability to support programs and services for older persons. The ratio of workers to retired persons will be considerably lower than it is today but the workers will be receiving higher wages/salaries and, even if they have to contribute greater proportions of wages to pay for Social Security and Medicare for their elders, they can still expect to be more affluent after deductions than workers today.

Family Structure

Because Baby Boomers had fewer children than their parents' generation, there will be fewer adult children to care for them if and when they require care. Offsetting this is the increase in multigenerational families and the expectancy that by the time the Baby Boomers reach retirement age, they will be members of four- or even five-generation families with an older generation of their parents but also with both adult children and grandchildren available to contribute to the family's well-being if necessary.

Although concern has been voiced about the future ratio of retirees to workers—the Dependency Ratio—and the fact that this seems likely to double, with fewer workers supporting more retirees, little attention has been given to the Total Dependency Ratio or the ratio of all non-working to all working people. This Total Dependency Ratio is not expected to increase because, whereas there are more retirees, there are also fewer children. This expectation is based on current numbers without taking into consideration any shifts in an immigrant population, which may swell the numbers of working persons. Although the U.S. may need to provide income subsidies and health and service support for more older persons in the future, this will coincide with a reduction in the provision of subsidies, services, and support to fewer children.

Children are a cost to society. They consume "an enormous quantity of resources without producing any" (Vladeck, 2001), so that having many children in a society is not good for the economy. "From a macroeconomic perspective, being older (as a country) is better than being younger" (Vladeck). However, in economic policy terms, children, as future adults, are needed to support our economic and intellectual property development.

Changes in Thinking about Retirement

The once "normal retirement age" of 65 is now obsolete. This age of eligibility for a pension was first identified by Bismarck in the 1880s and ensured that pension benefits would cost the Prussian government very little as few workers lived to that age at that time. Now that life expectancy has increased, it is time to "reformulate our vision of retirement age (perhaps beyond the already legislated move to 67 years) and reevaluate its implications for Social Security" (Vladeck, 2001). When Baby Boomers entered the labor force and were so numerous, employers had reason to encourage early retirement in older generations. Baby Boomers were better educated and more docile than their predecessors with less inclination to join unions. They were also younger and therefore cheaper to employ. As they age, and because this generation failed to replace itself in like numbers, employers may turn to incentives to keep persons in the work force beyond the usual retirement age.

Workers reaching 65 years of age may be more inclined than in the past to continue in the labor force. Data indicate that persons who have worked in physically stressful, inadequately remunerated jobs for most of their adult lives are eager to retire if they can be assured of an adequate income, whereas others are forced into retirement because of disability or illness. In the '70s and '80s of the twentieth century there was a gradual decline in the average retirement age of white collar and professional workers, fueled both by the eligibility to receive Social Security benefits at age 62, albeit at a reduced rate, and the interests of employers seeking to encourage retirement as a means of minimizing benefit costs. Since the 1990s this movement toward early retirement has faded. As workers remain healthy longer than ever before and are capable of working well into their seventies and eighties, they are opting to remain employed. The recent decline in the stock market is also encouraging middle-class workers to stay in the workplace as the equity they held in shares and stock options and were relying upon as retirement income has been severely depleted in the past two to three years. This phenomenon of delaying retirement, though not a desire or an option for all, is expected to continue as the Baby Boomers reach the age of potential retirement. Older persons staying in the work force augur well for Social Security and for the economy as a whole.

The federal government has already increased the age for receipt of full Social Security benefits by two years. This ratcheting up from 65 to 67 is a gradual process commencing in 2003 with annual age increments until the full age for eligibility of 67 is reached by 2027. However, increasing the minimum eligibility age for cash benefits in reality punishes the working class and the poor in health, who are forced into early retirement and have little or no savings to draw upon, while not contributing significantly to the already existing trend toward later retirement. The middle-class, more affluent workers tend to be indifferent to the change in eligibility age. States Vladeck (2001), "That means that it is bad social policy." [It suggests the] "importance of voluntary incentives to keep people in the workplace longer, rather than punitive measures that will have the greatest adverse effect on those with the least means."

Even without Vladeck's reframing of the Social Security crisis and the trends that can impact the program, there is considerable disagreement about its fiscal solvency. In 1997, it was anticipated that Social Security would face a shortfall as early as 2029. However, the Social Security Trustees' 2002 annual report noted that the fund will be able to pay all scheduled benefits until the year 2041, when the oldest Baby Boomers will be 94 years of age and the youngest will have already reached 77. This projection was made without factoring in future immigrants who, if their numbers remain the same as today, are expected to join the labor force and offset the numbers of retiring Baby Boomers, contributing Social Security taxes to the fund. If this occurs, the Social Security Trust Fund is likely to remain fully solvent until 2050 (Baker, 2002).

PLANNING FOR THE FUTURE

We no longer view retirement income as solely based on Social Security. Of equal importance is the role of retirement pensions, individual savings, and earnings from work. (The presence of health insurance is a vital, additional factor to be addressed in a later chapter.) Social Security is still with us and seems likely to continue its same role in the foreseeable future, although probably meeting fewer of our financial needs in retirement than it does today. The concept of supplementing Social Security with an employer pension, one's own personal investments and savings, and possibly continued wages, is now viewed as not only important but necessary (Rother, 2002).

Social Security and Pensions

Social Security was never intended to be an investment program. It is an insurance program, insuring income in retirement and covering survivors—spouses, children, and the disabled (Butler, 2001). However, current policy discussions at the federal level appear to view the program as an investment program, encouraging future beneficiaries to invest their Social Security payments in the private sector in lieu of the traditional wage-based taxes being placed into the Trust Fund. Management of the current system is efficient with only 0.7% of annual benefit payments required to administer the program. On the contrary, the monies that would be paid out to the financial industry to administer private accounts is estimated at 5%. There is also no protection for defined contributions handled in this manner and Baby Boomers would face the potential of lost contributions through risky investments.

Once a crucial element in an individual's savings for retirement years, 401(k) retirement plans have now fallen decisively in value. Such plans prove to be a good source of supplementing retirement monies but only if individuals actually invest the monies appropriately, experience good fortune, and leave the funds untouched. But as we have learned over this last year, with the accounting scandals and falsification of profits, there are risks that investors cannot readily anticipate. In addition, many companies provide their own stock as part of their employees' retirement savings and much of that stock has fallen dramatically in the past couple of years. Small employers have not been able to utilize the mechanism and there is also evidence that indicates that those earning below about twenty-five thousand a year do not put money into 401(k)s. This source of retirement savings is not an option for the lowest paid workers. Furthermore, many of those who do contribute to 401(k) plans choose to cash them out when changing jobs rather than roll them over into retirement savings (Butler, 2001; Rother, 2002).

Whether savings are in the form of 401(k)s, the purchase of bonds or stocks, or the maintenance of individual savings accounts, it has been recognized for many years that the American people are not saving enough for retirement years. A 1996 study conducted by AARP found that half of all workers were probably not saving enough and a third of all workers were not saving anything toward retirement (AARP, 1999). One third indicated that they would like to save but cannot afford to do so. Today, in 2004, with the downturn in the U.S. economy, the high unemployment rate, and poor performance of the stock markets, there is even less disposable income available for saving.

The policy of shifting the risks of saving for retirement to the individual can only result in some people being winners and some losers. This is contrary to the sense of social solidarity that existed when our systems were more inclusive. Substantial differences in wealth and income exist today within our older population and there is some evidence that even greater disparities in income will occur in the future. This is partly because of the shift in the private pension system from defined benefits to defined contributions. Those in the upper income levels during their working life will benefit more from the defined contributions system than they ever would have done under a defined benefits plan, whereas those at the lower level of earned income will be no better off and possibly far worse off as so many have no private pensions at all (Butler, 2001; Vladeck, 2001).

Work after Retirement

Finally, the role of work appears to be much more important in securing financial security in retirement than was generally believed. Currently, twenty percent of retirement income is from earnings, and this percentage is projected to grow.

For the individual retiree, the ability to continue to work (full- or part-time) in order to supplement income is becoming ever more important (Rother, 2002). The downturn in the economy is not only hampering each individual's opportunity to set aside income for retirement but is having a marked impact on older workers' decisions to retire. For many workers, their anticipated savings for retirement have been severely diminished over the last three to four years. This has led many to delay retirement and continue in the work force. A 2002 Gallup Poll of non-retired investors found a "major shift in retirement expectations" compared to four years earlier. Almost a fifth of the respondents said that they would delay their retirement by 4.4 years, and 83% said they would continue to "engage in work activities after reaching retirement age." At the same time, current retirees are reentering the work force, not only for personal satisfaction but for financial reasons, requiring the income to replace lost savings that had been counted on to supplement Social Security benefits.

It is impossible to predict the future state of the economy with any certainty, but it appears that the leading edge of the Baby Boomers will be facing a similar situation when they reach retirement age at the end of this decade. Many are already planning to continue working beyond the age of 65 years.

Living into the eighties and beyond is sometimes described as a woman's issue, as women tend to live longer than men and increasingly outnumber them as they grow older. This factor must be considered when discussing income security after retirement as women have fewer pensions and less savings income than men and are thus more apt to fall into poverty in their later years. This disparity occurs because women earn less than men; they frequently experience discontinuity of employment as they drop out of the labor force to raise children and provide caregiving for family members; there are no retirement benefits allowed for unpaid work in the home; and they have smaller pensions and can expect to outlive them. Given these factors "Social Security is the single most important financial resource for older women in the U.S." (AARP/ILC, 2003).

With the growing racial and ethnic diversity of the older population expected in the years ahead, it is important to recognize the inequalities in retirement security that currently exist between whites and people of color. A number of circumstances, similar to those experienced by women, converge to impact the ability of people of color to retire with sufficient income: "indicators which threaten the retirement security of people of color (are) low wages, intermittent work histories, family responsibilities, inadequate pension coverage, poor financial literacy, and discrimination" (Hudson, 2002, p. 1). This situation augurs badly for the economic well-being of the Baby Boom generation in its older years and suggests that the percent of poverty among this population will be considerable.

REFERENCES

AARP. (1999). Employee Benefits Research Institute. Retirement confidence survey, 1996. In *Boomers approaching midlife: How secure a future?* Washington, DC: AARP's Public Policy Institute.

AARP. (2002, May). *Beyond 50:02. A report to the nation on trends in health security.* Washington, DC: Author.

AARP/International Longevity Center. (2003). *Unjust desserts: Financial realities of older women.* Washington, DC: Author.

Baker, D. (2002, March 28). Social Security report kept from terrorists. *Social Security Information Project. Institute for America's Future.* Retrieved June 13, 2003 from http://socialsecurity.ourfuture.org

Butler, R. N. (2001, October 10). *Seven deadly issues.* Keynote address at Summit Meeting: *Can my eighties be like my fifties?* The New York Academy of Medicine, New York.

Gallup Poll. (2002). *Retirement revisited.* Conducted for UBS AG Financial Services Group.

Hudson, R. B. (2002, spring). People of color and the challenge of retirement security. *Public Policy and Aging Report, Gerontological Society of America.* Washington, D.C.

Purcell, P. J. (2001/2002). Pension sponsorship and participation: Trends and policy issues. *Social Security Bulletin, 64*(2), 93. Washington, DC: U.S. Government Printing Office.

Rother, J. (2002, October 25). *Respondent address.* Presentation at Third Summit Meeting. *Can my eighties be like my fifties?* The New York Academy of Medicine, New York.

Shalala, D. (2002, October 25). *Greying of America (and the world!). Keynote address.* Presentation at Third Summit Meeting. *Can my eighties be like my fifties?* The New York Academy of Medicine, New York.

Vladeck, B. (2001, October 10). *Keynote address.* Presentation at First Summit Meeting. *Can my eighties be like my fifties?* The New York Academy of Medicine, New York.

Chapter 5

Health Care Security: Medicare, Medicaid, Health Insurance, and Health Care Delivery

The single greatest threat to Boomers' economic security in retirement will be whether health costs continue to outpace incomes.

AARP, 1999

We must not allow our rendezvous with destiny to become a rendezvous with poverty and disease again.

Donna Shalala, 2002

INTRODUCTION

Health insurance, both private insurance and government programs, always has to be recognized as a factor of income security. A retiree may have sufficient income from Social Security, pensions, savings, and investments but if a large proportion of this is spent in paying for health care, all economic security is lost. Adequate health insurance has to be part of overall income security (Rother, 2002).

46

The government programs, Medicare and Medicaid, are already experiencing problems and having difficulties in keeping up with escalating health care costs. Increased premiums and reductions in coverage appear inevitable. These are programs that the majority of the American people pay into and rely upon to be there for them when they become eligible. They may be self-employed persons in their early sixties looking forward to becoming eligible for Medicare because they cannot afford private health insurance; working middle-class parents caring for a sick parent and raising children, paying bills with no excess monies to put aside for their retirement; or an elderly couple in poor health relying on Medicaid to cover their continually rising health costs.

By 2030, the Baby Boomers (double the number of today's aged) will all have reached 65 years of age and become eligible for Medicare under the existing regulations. As with Social Security, the size of Medicare expenditures will increase and, given the rising rates of health care costs, are likely to triple. The same models that show Medicare increasing from 2% to 6% of the Gross Domestic Product over the next forty years also show that real current dollar per capita income in the United States will increase between 50 and 100% over the same period of time. While this translates into increased income, the gain is likely to be offset by increased health care costs and a rising cost of living.

The cost of Medicaid has also grown substantially over the last twenty years, mainly because of the cost of long-term care for both the older frail population and the non-elderly disabled. Forty-four percent of people over the age of 85 have chronic health conditions, combined with disability and functional limitations. Currently, 11% of all those over 65 years of age fall into the over-85 range. By 2040 this percentage will have grown to 18%. As the size of this older population continues to grow, along with chronic illnesses, so will Medicaid costs.

HISTORY AND RATIONALE FOR MEDICARE

When the legislation was being enacted, one of the principal arguments on behalf of Medicare was that government would, through Medicare, assist middle-income, middle-aged families from total financial responsibility for caring for their aging parents, freeing these families to contribute their resources to finance higher education for their children. Caring for children was seen as a family responsibility that the advent of Medicare would help to maintain.

In 1965, shortly after Lyndon Johnson signed the act that established the Medicare program, Max Frankel of the *New York Times* approached the President and said, "My mother thanks you." "No," President Johnson replied. "It's you who should be thanking me." President Johnson's implication was that working people with families would no longer be forced to bankrupt their own savings and their dreams in order to provide for their parents and grandparents. Whereas today, at the beginning of the twenty-first century, few American families would be able to afford to send their children to college or to buy a house if Medicare and Social Security were nonexistent, this may not be true for much longer. By 2030, American families are likely to be contributing more for medical care of their parents' generation and paying more as well for higher education for their children. It may be time to renegotiate the deal between society and government, for it is imperative that we agree to continue and strengthen Medicare in ways that benefit all (Shalala, 2002).

RECENT CHANGES TO MEDICARE

During the eight years of the Clinton administration, work was begun to strengthen and alter Medicare in the following ways.

- The life of the Medicare Trust Fund was extended by at least three decades. The most massive crackdown on fraud and waste in the history of the program was initiated, resulting in over two billion dollars being returned to the Trust Fund.
- Legislation permitted people with disabilities to work and retain their Medicare for eight and a half years. Previously, disabled persons lost Medicare coverage on entering the work force, which reduced overall income for the majority and effectively dissuaded them from working.
- The management of Medicare was strengthened and the payment systems modernized, enabling Medicare payments within 16 days, faster than any HMO in the country.
- Prevention benefits were added. These included mammograms, bone density measurements, flu and pneumonia shots, colorectal cancer screenings, and glucose monitoring for diabetics. These new benefits are helping to prevent and detect diseases in their early stages when they are most treatable and simultaneously saving the costs of later-stage treatment (Shalala, 2002).

The Clinton Administration further proposed allowing the uninsured to buy into the Medicare system at age 55. The concept was to permit individuals to join this wider pool of health care insurance at that age at a reasonably priced premium that would be below what they would pay for health coverage in the open market. On officially entering the Medicare system at age 65, they would pay slightly more for their Medicare, making up the difference. This plan would fit well with the changing nature of today's employment market, with many of the 55–65 age group currently unemployed due to ill health or downsizing. Critics might argue that it would be the chronically ill, those unable to work, who would be most likely to buy into Medicare at an earlier age. This is probably true but exactly what is needed. The last thing we want, as a society, is large numbers of chronically ill, between the ages of 55 and 65, outside the health care system, getting sicker and sicker before reaching Medicare eligibility (Shalala, 2002).

The 2000 census counted 41 million Americans of all ages without health insurance for the year. If those who were without health insurance for part of the year were included, the total uninsured grew to almost 75 million persons. Most (78%) of today's uninsured come from working families, that is, families in which persons are employed full or part time or are actively seeking employment (Families USA Foundation, 2004). This situation has arisen because of temporary job loss, or the fact that not all jobs offer health insurance, or, if they do, workers cannot afford the high premiums. It is a sobering realization that one third to one half of all personal bankruptcies is due to the inability to pay medical bills.

FUTURE OF MEDICARE

Medicare is almost 40 years old. It needs to be reinvented. Medicare was originally conceptualized as employer-based acute care medical insurance. At the outset, it was strictly coverage of acute illness with no provision for coverage of preventive care, long-term care, or outpatient medications. Furthermore, it was principally oriented around the belief that the work force is made up of men, the sole breadwinners for the family. Society's trends and needs have changed in the intervening 35 years and it is time to restructure (Butler, 2002).

Though we have begun to restructure the Medicare system, we have so far failed to provide coverage for all. Whereas our focus here is on

Baby Boomers as the future U.S. older population, whatever we do as a nation in terms of health coverage has to be for all ages and must be intergenerational in nature. We have not accomplished universal health care, nor have we created a seamless system from employer–employee-based health care to Medicare, nor have we been able to provide guaranteed coverage of long-term care costs. Insurance companies are briskly offering long-term care insurance plans but, even with these plans, it is estimated that it will never be possible for more than 38% of Americans to afford the costs of long-term care (Weiner & Rivlin, 1998). Nor had we, until recently, found a way to cover prescription drugs via Medicare. When Medicare was created no one imagined either the role that prescription drugs would come to play in health care, especially in the lives of the old, chronically ill population (Butler, 2001; Shalala, 2002), or the impact that spiraling drug costs would have on the individual patient. As this book goes to press, legislation is being passed that includes limited coverage of prescription drugs, to take effect in 2006. There is some criticism of the bill, and it is too early to say whether it will remain in its current form.

In the interest of curbing the burgeoning costs of Medicare, the Federal government is seeking ways of holding down prices and containing costs. The Bush Administration favors privatization and is seeking ways for the Medicare eligible to enroll in health maintenance organizations (HMOs). The rationale is that the HMOs, while receiving reimbursement from the federal government, will keep overall costs down. To date, many HMOs have found the inclusion of Medicare-eligible consumers among their participants to be nonviable and several have pulled back from enrolling this population.

Medicare, and in fact all health insurance, needs to be transformed from a bill-paying program to a system that emphasizes prevention and cares for people as they grow older and require help in managing chronic illness. Dr. John Rother, Policy and Strategy Director for AARP, calls for Medicare to play a stronger part in moving our currently fragmented health care system into a more consumer/patient-oriented system with greater focus on delivery issues in the community setting (Rother, 2002).

Robert N. Butler, first Director of the National Institute on Aging, and currently Director of the International Longevity Center, agrees. Dr. Butler suggests that the restructuring of Medicare demands a move away from its current emphasis on acute care and hospitals, toward a major emphasis on care provided in the community. He envisages an entirely new structural basis and reorientation with teams of well-trained social workers, nurses, and physicians working together, paying attention to the entire spectrum of a continuum of care. Such a reorientation might even prove less costly than our current health care system with its focus on hospital care (Butler, 2001). The U.S. has the most expensive health care system in the world and yet has the means to change it and still provide quality care to all.

The two major problems besetting the U.S. health care system today are those of increasing costs beyond the rate of inflation and the fragmentation of services. The former contributes to increasing health insurance premiums and the growing number of persons without any health insurance who are effectively barred from receiving preventive health care. The latter problem of fragmentation leads to both over- and underutilization of health care. On one hand, the individual patient may be under the care of several physicians with little or no communication between them, resulting in duplication of diagnostic tests and interventions that may counteract each other. On the other hand, the same patient may receive care within one health care setting (nursing facility, hospital) and yet fail to receive appropriate ongoing care when discharged from the setting, due to lack of linkage between the settings. Older persons utilize health care to a greater degree than other age groups and are heavily impacted by these problems. Both Dr. Rother and Dr. Butler suggest that a major restructuring of Medicare and Medicaid by the government could result in a transformation of the U.S. health care system as a whole and be a means of controlling costs and overcoming fragmentation while simultaneously providing improved care.

HISTORY AND RATIONALE FOR MEDICAID

Medicaid legislation took place in 1965 when the provision of health care coverage for low-income individuals became part of the overall Social Security Act. Unlike Medicare, eligibility for Medicaid is not based on chronological age, but on category and income level. Popularly described as a program for "blind, disabled, and elderly," a Medicaid recipient must pass an income eligibility test and fall within one of these categories, or be a member of a single-parent family with dependent children. Medicaid covers 47 million low-income and disabled persons. Whereas Medicare is designed to meet acute health care costs, Medicaid has become the nation's major long-term care program, covering costs of nursing facility care or home care in the community as well as prescription drugs and the costs of acute care not covered by Medicare. The majority of beneficiaries today are poverty-level children or adults in families, but the bulk of expenditures go toward covering health care costs for elderly beneficiaries. As an older person covered under Medicare, one may also be eligible for Medicaid coverage if one meets the income eligibility standards.

Unlike Medicare, Medicaid is managed at the state level. The federal government sets minimum standards but the states are responsible for determining how income is calculated and the level of benefits to be covered. States also have the ability to extend coverage to additional services. Hence, the services that any one individual receives vary from state to state. With the advent of managed care and spread of health maintenance organizations (HMOs), Medicaid outlays were slowed in the early nineties when the number of Medicaid beneficiaries enrolled in managed care plans almost tripled. Eventually the efficiencies gained by managed care were outstripped by the increasing costs of medical care, and today HMOs are turning away from Medicaid enrollees, as they are from Medicare recipients, as being too expensive to handle.

FUTURE OF MEDICAID

The increase in the cost of covering Medicaid beneficiaries has had a dramatic impact on state governments and will continue to do so, especially if the federal government moves to block grants, shifting more of the total Medicaid costs to the state budgets. There is only one other category of expenditure that has grown more quickly for the states than Medicaid and this is the cost of correction departments. Research indicates that the net cost to society of incarceration in a state prison for one year is almost identical to the net cost of maintaining a person in a nursing home for the same period of time. Corrections is an industry that is largely focused on adolescent and post-adolescent males and, as such, carries hope for the future. Although the U.S. may have more older persons in need of long-term care in a nursing facility in the years ahead, it will also be supporting fewer persons in prison. The changing demography could allow government expenditures to be reallocated from corrections to Medicaid coverage of long-term care without a reduction in services to the prisoners who remain in the corrections system (Vladeck, 2001).

TRENDS IN HEALTH CARE COVERAGE

Most Americans who are not on Medicare or on Medicaid receive their health care insurance through an employer–employee-based system. Those who are forced to exit the workplace for health reasons may find themselves without coverage at a time when they need it most. The 1999 California Work and Health Survey (LaRock, 2001) found that nearly half of all California residents who retire early do so for health reasons. This population of early retirees is being joined by an increasing number of unemployed. No one anticipated that the economy at the beginning of the twenty-first century, and the nature of the job market would mean that large numbers of Americans who had worked all of their lives would find themselves without health care coverage, particularly between the ages of 55 and 65. We have talked a lot in this country about universal health care, especially in relation to coverage of children, but we have failed to recognize how employment itself has changed and is impacting health care coverage of adults, and Baby Boomers in particular. Even before the recent downturn in the economy, an increasing number of 50 to 64-year-olds were uninsured, with fewer employers at the beginning of the new century offering health care coverage to early retirees than they had ten years earlier. In 1993, 46% of large employers offered health insurance to their early retirees. By 2001, this had dropped to 29%. Included among the uninsured 50 to 64-year-olds are workers who have lost their jobs in the current downturn of our economy and the resulting downsizing (Shalala, 2002).

Even the employed are experiencing negative changes in health care coverage. The burden of health care coverage is increasingly shifting from employers to employees as health care costs continue to increase due to technological advances, a surge in biomedical research, and inefficiencies in the system. Contracting out for health coverage on the part of employers is resulting in higher costs to workers who are required to pay higher premiums for reduced coverage and more in copayments. Employers are moving toward defined contributions by paying a fixed amount per employee. In effect, only part of the employee-based system of today guarantees full health care benefits. The other part of the system covers only partial benefits and is increasingly adding requirements of what employees have to pay themselves in order to cover fully.

Similar trends are impacting the government-administered health care insurance for those over 65: Medicare. There is likely to be continuing debate over whether and how much money our government should guarantee to assure health care coverage under Medicare. One side of the political spectrum argues that the government ought to guarantee a certain amount of money, whereas the other side argues in favor of guaranteed benefits. To many, it seems preferable for the government to guarantee the benefits and for the debate to focus not on how much is guaranteed, but on exactly what the benefits will be. Medicare is already limited in its coverage. As a nation, we made a decision in 1965 that guaranteed Medicare would cover all expected health care costs within the defined parameters, not that the government would simply make a contribution. Today we are turning away from a defined benefit model to a defined contribution. There are those who argue in favor of defined contributions but this is likely to result in those who are becoming older, poorer, and sicker to be faced with covering more of the costs themselves (Rother, 2002; Shalala, 2002).

The recent experiences of the health maintenance organizations (HMOs) raises questions about our health care system, increasing the power of the argument that we need to move away from a guaranteed benefit system. The HMOs were working well while they had a very high percentage of healthy and younger persons on their registers. Once they started to enroll persons on Medicare, it became apparent that they could not keep their commitment to offer additional benefits at 95% of the costs of the fee for service. As we get older we suffer more ailments and become more expensive to carry within the system. Encouraging preventive measures among the Baby Boomers, tomorrow's older population, will lower these costs somewhat, but the oldest members of society will always be more costly to our health care system than the younger age groups (Shalala, 2002).

LACK OF PREPARATION FOR OUR FUTURE: WHAT IS NEEDED

Are the Baby Boomers prepared for their old age? Is society prepared? The answer to both these questions is a resounding No. Baby Boomers are not prepared financially, emotionally, or physically. As a society, we have not yet begun to plan seriously for the growing numbers of older persons among our ranks. Some of the areas on which we need to focus and to take action are the following.

Physical Activity

The U.S. is experiencing a national obesity epidemic. Over 50% of Americans are overweight, and this includes Baby Boomers. Even 20%

of America's children are obese. We are the fattest nation in the world. Obesity is leading to an increase in "old age diabetes," Type II diabetes, even among 10-year-old children (Butler, 2001).

Rather than deploring obesity, it is more appropriate not only to reduce our consumption of fast foods but to focus on physical activity. Lack of activity is the major cause of the problem. Most Americans are not physically active. They do not walk. The solution to our sedentary life style is to become a nation of walkers. If one walks 10,000 steps a day, one's weight is maintained. If one walks more than 10,000 steps—13, 14, or 15,000—one loses weight. AARP is working with the Robert Wood Johnson Foundation to develop a strong pro-physical activity program in the cities of Madison, Wisconsin, and Richmond, Virginia. The goal is to mobilize Baby Boomers and older people to become more physically active on a regular basis through walking those ten thousand steps daily (Butler, 2001).

Long-Term Care

There is insufficient attention at the federal level to long-term care and the anticipated future increase in chronically ill older persons who will require both medical care and assistance with activities of daily living. At the national and local levels, there is a desire to maintain this frail older population in their own homes with needed services provided within the community. As a society we need to reframe the health care system to allow this to happen. This will include determining the levels of caregiving responsibilities on the part of the informal system (family and friends) and the formal system, and developing partnerships that integrate the two systems to provide quality care.

Quality care of our chronically ill and disabled elderly is possibly the major challenge facing our health care system in the twenty-first century. Most Baby Boomers will face an extended period of managing chronic illness or disability, although it is forecast that only a small percentage will be functionally disabled. The existing health care system is not set up to manage chronic illness well but we do know what works and needs to be done. We do know that putting people together in support groups, involving the chronically ill person and the family in the care arrangement, delivering care via a team of providers (most frequently a physician, nurse, and social worker), and establishing continuing relationships between the chronically ill or disabled person and the health care providers do work. Organizing to make system-wide changes to adopt these practices is a necessary step toward providing quality care to the chronically ill elders in our future.

Research

Continued research is needed on age-related diseases and conditions. For instance, there is substantial ongoing research on Alzheimer's disease but we are far from a solution. We know very little about the central nervous system, its function and pathology. We anticipate that there will be as many as 14 million people with Alzheimer's disease by 2040. The cost of caring for this population will be enormous.

There has been a growth in recent years in what is referred to as longevity medicine and science, with researchers seeking to understand the biology of longevity and to find ways of extending the normal human life span. One means of doing this may be via embryonic stem cell technology, which eventually may allow us to repair or replace diseased and malfunctioning organs. Such research is controversial and currently unsupported federally in the U.S. but it offers hope for the cure of many age-related diseases (e.g., macular degeneration, Alzheimer's, and Parkinson's disease). Regenerative medicine, which may become one of the most important medical areas of the twenty-first century, is developing overseas.

The practice of gene-based medicine will characterize future medical care, enabling individuals and families to gain understanding of their disease prospects, what the pathological proteins created by the genes might result in, and how those proteins might be neutralized. Gene therapy can prevent or change a disease based on a defective gene, annihilating its impact on the body. It is not too idealistic to imagine a future in which these advances in our understanding of diseases and physical malfunctioning will transform our health in later years, although the financial cost to society and the individual may be huge (Butler, 2001).

Education, Training, and Recruitment

Health care professionals require education and training in care of the older person. Medicare provides 6.2 billion dollars annually for education but most of this resource is devoted to training of residents in areas other than geriatrics. Although this is commendable, no Medicare funds are set aside for the development of educators within our 145 allopathic and osteopathic schools of medicine. The Health Resources and Services Administration funds Geriatric Education Centers that provide continuing education to all health care professionals, including physicians, and administers the Geriatric Academic Career Award. There are also private entities, such as the John A. Hartford Foundation, that support geriatric education in medical, nursing, and social work schools for a selected number of students and the development of faculty with a focus on aging. However, much more is needed. It is vital that funds be made available for the training of educators in the care of the elderly. The U.S. demographics indicates that whatever their chosen specialty, physicians, nurses, and social workers will all find, on entering the work force, that a significant proportion of their clients and patients are older persons. If there are teachers, then no one will graduate from medical school or residency programs, nursing or social work schools, without exposure to knowledge about older people.

We are faced with a shortage of nurses and social workers in this country so not only do we need to train educators to pass on knowledge of care for the elderly, but we also need to attract more individuals into nursing and social work through increased salaries and better working conditions (Butler, 2001).

Educated Consumers

Baby Boomers are better informed about their health care than their parents' generation but as a group, all members need to become informed users of health care. Although the health care system is fragmented, there is still more information available to consumers than ever before, both in terms of public information about health conditions and treatment options and information on quality of health care provided by organizations and individuals. This trend toward making medical information available and encouraging patients to become partners in management of their own health care has been spurred by the patient rights movement and is growing in power.

It is recognized that one factor determining how patients fare within the system is their attitude and approach toward health care. Searching out information, becoming a partner with one's doctor, and being discriminatory in making treatment decisions based on quality of care makes a difference. If Baby Boomers, as a group, were to be proactive in this manner, it would also make a substantial difference to the entire system, driving it in the right direction and generating health care reform (Rother, 2002).

SUMMARY

Baby Boomers want to be assured that Social Security, Medicare, and Medicaid remain in place and viable for their future.

Social Security and Medicare have been called the "Third Rail" in American politics and, as such, are viewed as indispensable rights. This "Third Rail" is currently under siege and unless we act to restructure these programs we will fall backward in our social contract with the American population. "If we fail to protect and enhance and change our programs appropriately . . . our failure will be dramatic." We ought not to nor can we give our seniors and our disabled and our future seniors and disabled less security and freedom than they have now. "We must not allow our rendezvous with destiny to become a rendezvous with poverty and with disease again" (Shalala, 2002). In order to avoid this, we must not be afraid of improving and expanding the programs. Our older, frail members of society will always be a costly population in terms of health coverage and care but we cannot turn away from them. Creative solutions can be found by building new partnerships among businesses, families, religious and community organizations, schools, and the health and medical communities (Shalala, 2002). Social Security needs to be more generous and more distributive in the future to compensate for the anticipated reduction in income for lower and middle wage earners from private pension plans. Race, class, and national origin will become central to these issues of social and economic policy and must be factored into all our deliberations (Vladeck, 2001).

The question being asked by government and across the country is: Can we afford to maintain and expand our fundamental commitments to older Americans? According to Vladeck (2001), the "crisis" in Social Security and Medicare is a "rhetorical crisis . . . not a real one," a political rather than an economic phenomenon. Whether we can continue to afford adequate income and health care benefits to persons over 65 is not a challenging question. The more pertinent question is what kind of society and ideals do we want thirty years from now? The way we answer this will define our society in the decades ahead. If we wish to secure these programs and honor our commitment to all age groups, we must act now and begin restructuring for the future. This is both morally sound and financially feasible. "We can if we want to" (Vladeck, 2001).

REFERENCES

Butler, R. N. (2001, October 10). *Seven deadly issues.* Keynote address at Summit Meeting: *Can my eighties be like my fifties?* The New York Academy of Medicine, New York, NY.

Families. (2003, March). *USA Report.*

Families USA Foundation. (2004). One in three; Non-elderly Americans without health insurance, 2002–2003. Report 1-44. Publication No. 04-104. Washington, D.C.

LaRock, S. (2001). Few Boomers will choose freedom to work allowed by new law. *Aging Today,* January/February. Vol. XXII, No. 1.

Rother, J. (2002, October 25). *Respondent address.* Presentation at Third Summit Meeting. *Can my eighties be like my fifties?* The New York Academy of Medicine, New York, NY.

Shalala, D. (2002, October 25). *Greying of America (and the world!).* Keynote Address Presentation at Third Summit Meeting: *Can my eighties be like my fifties?* The New York Academy of Medicine, New York, NY.

Vladeck, B. (2001, October 10). *Keynote address.* Presentation at First Summit Meeting: *Can my eighties be like my fifties?* The New York Academy of Medicine, New York, NY.

Weiner, J. M., & Rivlin, A. M. (1998). *Caring for the disabled elderly. Who will pay?* Washington, DC: National Academy Press.

Chapter 6

Long-Term Care: Who Will Care for Us?

INTRODUCTION

As Americans live longer, they are also living longer with chronic illnesses and diseases. Geriatricians are fond of saying, "If you live long enough, you will be sure to get cancer" or Alzheimer's, arthritis, or another age-related disease. But they are right. The longer we live, the more likely it becomes that we will encounter one or more age-related diseases and/or conditions, such as diminished sight or hearing. For example, about 58% of all those over the age of 70 report having arthritis although this does not necessarily mean that they are disabled by it (Centers for Disease Control and Prevention, 1999). The Baby Boomers are no exception and can anticipate living even longer than their parents' generation, with perhaps an even greater chance of experiencing some part of their old age living with ongoing health-impaired conditions that require continuing care.

Recognition of the increasing life expectancy in the United States and the fact that many older persons can anticipate experiencing chronic illness over a number of years is resulting in a focus on long-term care needs. In spite of this shift in thinking, the health care system is still organized around an acute care model. The demand for long-term care, maintaining an individual's functioning rather than curing, has given rise to the belief that long-term care is best provided in the community. Older persons prefer to remain at home and generally fare better in their home environment and familiar surroundings. Advocates for home care argue that provision of services in the community is less costly in terms of public monies. Residential nursing facilities are viewed as most appropriate for those who require 24-hour nursing care as well as for short-term patients undergoing a few weeks of rehabilitation before returning to their homes. Meanwhile, many older persons with disabilities live in their own homes in the community, and while not in need of full-time institutional care are in need of some care. However, while the trend of nursing facilities to accept the most disabled continues, the "supply of home and community-based services for others in need of long-term care has not increased concomitantly" (Vladeck, 1998). The Olmstead decision (Olmstead: 527 U.S. 581, 1999) of 1999 determined that the Americans with Disabilities Act (ADA) may *require* states to provide community-based services rather than institutional placements for people with disabilities but it is too soon to judge whether this determination will result in a substantial increase in community-based care for older persons.

ANTICIPATED REALITY: LIVING WITH CHRONIC CONDITIONS

In general, today's older individuals enjoy a period of good health and activity from retirement until their late seventies. At this stage, their health begins to be compromised as age-related diseases appear and chronic conditions worsen, leading to an increased reliance on the health care system. By the time they reach their mid-eighties, many, but certainly not the majority, are becoming functionally impaired, require assistance to remain living in the community, and perhaps even require help with activities of daily living (ADLs).* The greatest fear of older Americans with disabilities is that they will lose their independence (AARP, 2003).

---

*Activities of Daily Living (ADLs) and Instrumental Activities of Daily Living (IADLs): As a means of measuring functional disability, health care professionals and researchers assess an individual's ability to perform *activities of daily living* such as bathing, dressing, eating, getting in or out of bed or a chair, using the toilet, and getting around inside the home, and *instrumental activities of daily living* or ability to manage one's own affairs including grocery shopping, preparing meals, managing money, using the telephone, taking medications, and getting around outside the home. A three-point scale is utilized to indicate whether an individual is unable to perform, able to perform with assistance, or able to perform independently.

The situation is not all bleak. The rate of disability in those over 65 years of age has declined by 25% over the last twenty years (Manton & Gu, 2001). Only one third of all those over 65 report that they are handicapped from one or more chronic conditions (Administration on Aging, 2001). Most of this one third is found among those over 85 years old. Within this group of old-old persons, 57% need assistance with one or more instrumental activities of daily living (IADLs)* and 44% are "living simultaneously with chronic illness, disability, and limitations in daily functioning" (AARP, 2003), but this also means that 43% of those over 85 remain functionally independent, cognitively and physically intact. Those who do require assistance rely on family, friends, and/or the formal care system to help them.

The Baby Boomer generation may find that its active early years of aging extend further into its early eighties and that many can expect to live into their nineties and beyond. As the Boomers' rendezvous with chronic illness and poor health may be delayed, they may live long enough to catch up and experience similar needs for long-term care as their parents do today at an earlier age. The good news for Baby Boomers is that as people age, the physical environment and social network are the most important determinants in an individual's ability to remain living independently at home. The rate of disability among the older population is declining. This trend may well continue, enabling an increasingly larger percentage of the future older population to remain free of disability even into their nineties and beyond and even while dealing with chronic health conditions, especially if they live in a safe environment with a supportive network. A recent AARP survey concludes that as people age, their "physical environment and social network can make or break" their chance of remaining independent (AARP, 2003).

INTO THE FUTURE

From all reports, the Baby Boomers do not consider the aging of their generation and the potential for disability. Old age is not for them, as witnessed by the emphasis on remaining young and the popularity of treatments designed to keep the body youthful. Practicing good nutritional habits, exercising, and not smoking will physically prepare many Baby Boomers for old age to a greater degree than their parents and enable them to live longer and more actively even with chronic health difficulties. But in spite of society's emphasis on prevention, too few of this generation are practicing or benefiting from such measures. The rate of obesity is rising in the U.S., as are the rates of diabetes and heart disease that accompany it.

This lack of prevention may be linked to denial of any future that might include illness and potential disability. When they do look ahead, Baby Boomers know that they do not wish to grow old in the same way as their parents and grandparents. They envisage a healthy, active life pursuing their interests, with a large network of friends growing old and wise alongside them. If they do consider what their lives at 80 years of age may be, the wish-image that presents itself is of living in their own housing, which is "architecturally and environmentally acceptable, with easy access to a variety of programs and services and opportunities for service to others, learning, travel and personal and spiritual growth." They foresee this lifestyle as enabled by a system of public and private partnerships within the community. If they should become disabled and functionally impaired, they will remain at home, being cared for by family, friends, and/or formal caregivers who share similar backgrounds and interests (Group discussion, Summit #1).

WHO WILL CARE FOR THE FRAIL?

Baby Boomers gave birth to fewer children than their parents' generation did. This decline in the fertility rate has continued until today, the U.S. total fertility rate is 2.034, below the replacement rate (National Center for Health Statistics, 2003). Will the Baby Boomers have adult children available and prepared to care for them if they become frail and in need of care? This is a concern of demographers and sociologists, even if the Baby Boomers themselves have failed to ask the question. A similar concern is voiced over the availability of formal caregivers—paid home-care workers, home attendants, companions—who might be expected to fill the caregiving gaps when family members are not available. Traditionally, those who work in these jobs are among the lowest paid and least skilled members of the labor force, and it is frequently recent immigrants who fill these positions, often as the means of starting up the employment ladder en route to realizing the American dream. In latter years, the U.S. immigration policy has hardened, and fewer people are being welcomed into the country as legal immigrants, although the long-term projection is for continued growth. The U.S. population, now at 292 million, is expected to increase to 420 million by 2050, with much of the increase resulting from immigration (McFalls, 2003).

CAREGIVERS OF TODAY

A look at today's caregivers will inform our planning for the future. Currently, 85% of the care needs of our older population is provided by family and friends—the informal caregivers. Approximately 25 million family caregivers provide some assistance to an older relative; about 6–9 million of those provide daily assistance with personal care or activities of daily living (ADLs) (Noelker, 2001). In monetary terms, this is translated into an economic value of $196 billion (Arno, Levine, & Memmott, 1999). Most often the caregiver is a family member, usually an adult child, followed by spouses, and then siblings. There is even a term coined to describe this group of adult children—*the Sandwich Generation*—which acknowledges that the adult children are frequently caught in the middle, pressured with providing care to generations on either side, to their own children and to their parents. On average, a woman in the U.S. spends 17 years caring for children and 18 years caring for elderly parents (U.S. Department of Labor, 2000). Caregiving is still largely seen as the responsibility of women so that it tends to be the daughter or daughter-in-law who provides the hands-on-care. In terms of the caregiving spouse, it is generally the wife who cares for the husband. The female usually outlives the male, and when her turn comes to receive care, her husband is frequently not available and she must turn to her adult children. Caregiving may involve a few hours weekly but may also mean the provision of twenty-four hour care, depending on the level of need.

Caring for an older relative or friend in poor health is enormously stressful, even if the responsibility is willingly and lovingly undertaken, as it most often is. There may be financial stress due to coverage of health costs and, frequently, the loss of income as the result of the caregiver dropping out of the labor force in order to provide care. There is physical stress involved in nursing a frail, older person who requires assistance in bathing and toileting. Older caregivers—spouses, siblings, or friends—are especially vulnerable to this physical stress as they themselves may also be older persons with health problems of their own. Above all, caregivers identify emotional stress as the most difficult aspect of providing care for a relative or close friend. Former relationships are changed with the dependency of the individual receiving care and, alongside love, the caregiver tends to experience frustration, hopelessness, and anger, which are then compounded by guilt for feeling these emotions. There are numerous studies concerning caregivers' stress and mental health, leading researchers and mental health workers to emphasize the need to focus on the caregivers' well-being as well as that of the care recipient. Caregivers' stress is related to the number of persons who share the caregiving responsibilities. A family in which there are several persons to share the responsibilities of caring is likely to feel less stress than the family in which the caring responsibility falls to one or two persons—an argument, perhaps, for large family networks.

Considerable attention has been given to ethnic and cultural differences in caring for older family members. Latino and African-American families hold a more recent past than whites in which older relatives were members of large familial networks and were cared for when frail as a natural part of family life. Three-generational households, in which the grandparents helped raise the grandchildren and which expedited reciprocal caring when this was needed, were the norm. Immigrant populations, from a variety of cultural backgrounds, observe that American families do not hold the same commitment to their elderly as is found in their home countries, but establish separate households and tend to view caring for frail parents as a chore. There remains debate as to whether this perspective is valid or whether the differences between ethnic groups are caused less by culture than by a shift from an agricultural to an industrialized society and an economy that has permitted the separation of households within the extended family unit. A study during the 1990s of New York City elderly and the care and assistance they receive found that Latino elderly had the most frequent face-to-face contact with their children compared to African Americans or whites. Seventy-nine percent of Latino elderly saw at least one child each week compared with 75% of African-American elderly and 60% of white elderly. Despite this difference, all three groups were in close contact with adult children and received assistance when it was needed. Two thirds of all adult children had regular in-person contact with their parents and one fourth spoke to their parents in-person or by phone every day. Given the increased cultural diversity among older persons expected in the future, we must take care that a belief in a cultural foundation for family caregiving is not used to justify an absence or reduction in formal services provided by the government to assist family caregivers.

Among all ethnic groups in the U.S., there are adult children who are at a distance, having relocated in search of work opportunities, and older persons who have moved in retirement, in search of warmer climates and easier life styles. This means that caregiving at a distance is a common phenomenon, which carries its own stresses and a shift in the nature of the caregiving tasks.

CAREGIVING TOMORROW

As the huge amount of care provided by family members testifies, most older persons can depend on their families to provide care for as long as they are able. But not all older persons have families. Some may be from disconnected families whose members do not expect or wish to help each other, but most are those who never married or had children. In the future, given the declining birth rate, many Baby Boomers may find that they enter old age without adult children available to assist them. A further question must be asked: Even if there are adult children available, will they be willing to shoulder caregiving responsibilities or, perhaps more pertinent, will their parents want them to do so? Baby Boomers attending the Summit meetings made it clear that whereas they wanted a future in which they were in contact with their children, they did not necessarily expect or want these adult children to be responsible for their care over long periods of time. Similar attitudes have been identified by studies that have shown that though the parents of the Baby Boomers cared for their own parents as needed, they, perhaps because of their own experience, did not want their children, the Baby Boomers, to shoulder the same responsibilities. It seems that the Boomers are now saying the same to their children, that is, I am doing it but I don't want you to do it.

The changing family structures that we are witnessing today may be the solution for long-term care of our older population in the future. Divorce, single parenthood, remarriage, the increase in step-families, same-sex partners, adoption have all broadened our perception of family, so that although the stereotypical "two parent, two point five children" family still exists, there is enormous variation. Family networks, including persons of all ages, connected in a variety of ways, are commonplace. Optimists view these trends as meaning that there will be more adult relatives and friends to provide assistance; pessimists see only a weakening of close familial ties, meaning fewer available to help.

LONG-TERM CARE AND FORMAL CAREGIVERS

Although the extent and availability of informal caregivers in the future to provide long-term care is uncertain, it is evident that an increase in the formal caregivers, whether paid by private or public monies, is a necessity. Nursing facilities are already understaffed and there is a scarcity of formal caregivers to provide care in the community. A recent report to Congress released by the National Institutes of Health states that the U.S. will need three times as many long-term care workers as are now employed to meet the care needs of the Baby Boom generation (NIH, 2003). This is an increase from the 1.9 million employed in 2000 to approximately 5.7–6.5 million. Currently the ratio of home care workers to those requiring home care is one to seven. It is estimated that by 2050 the ratio will be closer to one to twenty-four. Meanwhile, inadequate staffing and lack of supervision are among the causes of poor nursing home care (Kayser-Jones et al., 2003).

Paraprofessionals such as nursing assistants, home-care aides, and personal care workers and attendants are poorly paid with few if any benefits, receive minimum training, and have few opportunities for career advancement. The work fails to attract or retain workers, who tend to find employment elsewhere. The "typical paraprofessional worker is a middle-aged, single mother with a low level of educational attainment, living below or just above the poverty line" (Stone, 2001). To offset the constant shortage of workers, the industry relies on immigrants, low wage earners from underdeveloped countries, who find that entering the long-term care field is a means of securing a foothold in the job market. Vladeck (2001) asks whether by perpetuating this exploitation of immigrant workers we are, as a society, supporting our old population at the expense of the young in less developed countries? Aside from this ethical quandary, it is practical to ask, given the numbers of old people that we anticipate will need long-term care in the future, whether there will be an increased flow of immigrants to this country in sufficient numbers. Projections suggest that the numbers of anticipated immigrants will be partially responsible for increasing the U.S. population by 130 million between today and 2050 (McFalls, 2003). However, unless nursing facility and home care work conditions are vastly improved, it will be difficult to attract sufficient numbers of long-term care workers into the field.

FINANCING LONG-TERM CARE:
PUBLIC AND PRIVATE MEANS

Today, the average cost of long-term care in institutionalized settings such as nursing facilities is estimated at about $55,000 per year. Medicare covers a limited number of days following hospitalization, but few individuals and their families can afford the expense of a nursing facility for more than a few months once the Medicare coverage ceases. Medicaid has therefore become the main financier of nursing facility care. Medicaid is an income tested program available to those with very low annual incomes. Once individuals have depleted their resources in covering the cost of care, they can become Medicaid eligible and the cost is picked up by the government. If formal long-term care is provided in the home setting in the community, Medicare will currently cover the cost of a limited number of home care days but when this coverage ends, the individual must once again pick up the costs or, if deemed eligible, turn to Medicaid. If ineligible, older persons must meet the expenses of care out of their own income and savings, often at great cost. It has been estimated that no more than 38% of Americans will ever be able to afford the costs of long-term care (Weiner & Rivlin, 1998). To add to the difficulties of meeting the costs of health care is the finding that consumers of long-term care services and their families are generally confused as to what Medicare will offer. Medicare is an important source of coverage for beneficiaries who need skilled care (Center for Medicare Education, 2003) but does not provide comprehensive long-term care coverage by any means.

In 1999, the U.S. spent an approximate total of $134 billion on long-term care, two thirds of which was for nursing facility care and the other third for home care. Chen (2003) notes that the majority of these costs are mostly covered by the individual out of income and savings and by public monies (Medicare, Medicaid), with insurance policies contributing only a small share of the total. This situation is unlikely to be sustainable because it tends to impoverish many people and thereby severely strains Medicaid budgets nationwide. Indeed, the current beleaguered status of both the Medicare and Medicaid funds makes it appear unlikely that these programs will be able to sustain coverage of long-term care in a future in which the number of individuals requiring long-term care is expected to be much greater and more costly than it is today.

Much of the federal and national debate over health care focuses on the future of Medicare and Medicaid and what changes are required to assure their solvency. Whatever alterations are made to these programs, it is clear that the future financing of long-term care must be a public-private partnership. Health insurance companies perceive a market for long-term care insurance and are actively promoting insurance programs that will meet future needs. As to be expected, annual premiums vary greatly, depending on the age at time of purchase and type of coverage desired. Purchasing long-term care insurance before the age of 50 can cost less than a thousand dollars annually but may rise to $5–6,000 per year if purchased in one's late seventies (AARP, 2003). Given that the odds of requiring extensive long-term care for any one individual are fairly low, and the fact that the Baby Boom generation is failing to plan for its old age, it is not surprising that sales of long-term care private insurance have been low, contributing to the high premiums. For most individuals, the time of facing the possibility of needed long-term care is post-retirement, when chronic illnesses may already be evident, by which time the premiums are at their highest while annual income may be substantially lower than it was during pre-retirement years.

Currently, the Baby Boomers are not sure whether long-term care insurance is worthwhile and a wise investment. If they do have income to invest, in general they will opt for securing these monies in private investments and savings that are not lost if long-term care is not required. *Consumer Reports* took a look at long-term care insurance in 2003 and noted that long-term-care insurance is an expensive form of insurance and if one purchases it early at the lower premiums, one may not need it for 30 or 40 years if at all. Meanwhile the premiums add up and may exceed higher premiums paid at older ages and over fewer years (*Consumer Reports*, 2003). The report's guidelines are to "skip a plan if your net worth is less than $200,000 . . . or your assets exceed $1.5 million . . . or you can't afford the premiums for the necessary coverage, or you don't anticipate having enough money to cover sharp premium hikes that may take place during the years you own the policy." On the other hand, consider a plan if you have a chronic health condition and are about 55 years of age, if your assets are between $200,000 and $1.5

million and you must protect them for family members, or if you have
no one who will be available to take care of you at home (*Consumer
Reports*, 2003). Insurance companies aim to sign up a large proportion
of the U.S. population for long-term care insurance, which will result
in lower, more affordable premiums. In the absence of this, the Federal
government and the insurance companies need to fashion a partnership
in which all are covered and the financial risks are shared, perhaps
through government payment of insurance premiums for low income
individuals and tax incentives.

POLICIES FOR THE FUTURE: LONG-TERM CARE IN THE COMMUNITY

Government policy is in favor of long-term care at home, in the community—witness the Olmstead decision. As long as there are older persons
who need 24-hour nursing care beyond the capacity of the family and
community resources to provide, and as long as there are those without
family or support network of any kind, nursing facilities will be required.
For all others, long-term care in the community is the ideal, not just
because it costs less for the government to cover but also because it is
widely accepted that older persons in need of long-term care generally
do better if they remain in their own familiar setting. In 1999 Robert
Kane warned that "it is high time that medical care addressed its anach-
ronistic behavior. . . . The best (long term) care is that which avoids
exacerbations that are associated with dramatic interventions and high
cost. The primary goal of such care is controlling disease rather than
curing it."

If, as a country, we are opting for care in the home above all else,
the policies we favor must be those that make long-term care at the
community level accessible and available, and assist the informal caregivers—family and friends—in their role. The Summit presenters, as well
as Baby Boomers who had or were providing family care to an elderly
parent or relative, had several suggestions.

- Reframe caregiving as a community and family issue in which
  formal caregivers from within the community and family and
  friends work together. The older person, family members, and/
  or friends should be essential members of the health care team
  in what Dr. Ronald Adelman (Adelman, 2002) termed a "patient/
  consumer centered team."

- Develop public/private partnerships in order to assure accessible, affordable services (e.g., state-wide cooperatives in which health care systems, insurance companies, and state departments join to create available and affordable long-term care services).
- Collaborate with younger, disabled populations and service systems to maximize resources and contain costs.
- Create family allowances to defray costs of caregiving and enable the older person and/or family to purchase long-term care services either from a formal agency or from a family member or friend.
- Time spent out of the labor force in providing unpaid long-term care should be counted as work hours for Social Security purposes.
- Make provisions in the workplace for employees with long-term caregiving responsibilities—flexible hours, shared-time jobs, continued health care benefits.
- Develop senior caregivers, either paid or volunteers with stipends.
- Promote "family networks" through tax deductions in which all members contribute to care of those in need, either in monies to enable purchase of care or in kind, the provision of caregiving hours.

Many of the proposed policies and programs acknowledge consumer partnership and direction. Interest in health care consumers' right to make decisions about their own care has led to a growing movement in favor of consumer involvement in the delivery of long-term health care. "Consumer direction in long-term care starts with the premise that individuals with long-term care needs should be empowered to make decisions about the care they receive, including having primary control over the nature of the services and who, when, and how the services are delivered" (Stone, 2000, p. 5). Consumer-directed care is a radical departure from the norm as it focuses on a non-medical approach, assigning the medical profession to membership within an interdisciplinary team and placing the consumer in control. Baby Boomers participating in the Summits expressed their support of this growing movement, which is echoed in the above suggestions.

The need for long-term care will continue to be a priority throughout the first half of this century. Some of the suggested innovations are already being tested. For example, Boston College has demonstrated the success of a program in which disabled Medicaid beneficiaries direct their own care, receiving monetary allocations that they use to purchase care from family, friends, or formal agencies. Unmet needs for care

are reduced and the quality of life of the program participants is improved. The Robert Wood Johnson Foundation is currently underwriting the cost of replicating this program in several states (Program offers new models, 2004).

Some of the above suggestions by the Baby Boomers are easy to establish within individual families, whereas others require major policy shifts. Baby Boomers would be wise to acknowledge the existence of potential frailty and chronic illness in their later years and to plan ahead for such contingencies. As a society, the steps we take to assure available, accessible, quality care from formal caregiving agencies that partner with and are supportive of the informal caregiving system of family and friends, will be a measure of the regard in which we hold our elders.

REFERENCES

AARP. (2003, April). Beyond 50:03. A report to the nation on independent living and disability. AARP's Public Policy Institute.

Adelman, R. (2002, April 24). Presentation at Second Summit Meeting: *Can my eighties be like my fifties?* The New York Academy of Medicine, New York, NY.

Administration on Aging. (2001). Profile of older Americans, 2000. http://www.aoa.gov/aoa/STATS/profile/default.htm

Arno, P., Levine, C., & Memmott, M. (1999). The economic value of informal caregiving. *Health Affairs, 18*(2), 182–188.

Center for Medicare Education. (2003). *Medicare and long-term care.* Washington, DC: *Issue Brief,* Vol. 4, No. 4.

Centers for Disease Control and Prevention. (1999). *Targeting arthritis: The nation's leading cause of disability.* Washington, DC.

Chen, Y. (2003). Funding long-term care: Applications of the trade-off principle in both public and private sectors. *Journal of Aging and Health, 15*(1), 15–44.

Consumer reports. (2003, November). Do you need long-term-care insurance? Yonkers, NY: Consumer Union of the U.S., Inc.

Kane, R. L. (1999). A new model of chronic care. *Generations, Integration of Care in a Changing Environment, XXIII*(2), 35–37.

Kayser-Jones, J., Schell, E., Lyons, W., Kris, A., Chan, J., & Beard, R. (2003). Factors that influence end-of-life care in nursing homes: The physical environment, inadequate staffing and lack of supervision. *Gerontologist, 43*(Special Issue II), 76–84.

McFalls, J., Jr. (2003). *Population Bulletin, 58*(4). (Electronic version). Population Reference Bureau. Retrieved 1/22/04 from www.prb.org/Template.cfm?Section=PRB&template=/ContentManagement/ContentDisplay.cfm&ContentID9789

National Center for Health Statistics. (2003). As referenced on Population Reference Bureau website. Retrieved 1/22/04 from www.prb.org/Template.cfm?

Section=PRB&template=/ContentManagement/ContentDisplay.cfm&Content
ID9527

National Institutes of Health. (2003). *Report to Congress* (Electronic version). Retrieved 11/30/03 from http://aspe.hhs.gov/daltcp/reports/Hcwork.pdf

Noelker, L. S. (2001). The backbone of the long-term-care workforce. *Generations, Journal of the American Society on Aging, XXII*(1), 85–91.

Olmstead: 527 U.S. 581, 1999. Americans with Disabilities Act/Olmstead Decision. Centers for Medicare and Medicaid Services. http://www.cms.hhs.gov/olmstead

Program offers new models for care of the elderly and disabled: $7M grant boosts Boston College Graduate School of Social Work study. (2004, January 22). *The Boston College Chronicle.* See also Robert Wood Johnson Foundation website, www.rwjf.org

Stone, R. I. (2000). Introduction: Consumer direction in long-term care. *Generations, Journal of the American Society on Aging, XXIV*(3), 5–9.

Stone, R. I. (2001). Research on frontline workers in long-term care. *Generations, Journal of the American Society on Aging, XXV*(1), 49–57.

U.S. Department of Labor. (2000). Balancing caregiving and work. Study commissioned by the U.S. House of Representatives.

Vladeck, B. (1998, June 16). *The future of long-term care.* Presentation at the Long-Term Care Planning Symposium, Mount Sinai Health Care Foundation, Cleveland, OH, pp. 3–4.

Vladeck, B. (2001, October 10). *Keynote address.* Presentation at First Summit Meeting: *Can my eighties be like my fifties?* The New York Academy of Medicine, New York.

Weiner, J. M., & Rivlin, A. M. (1988). *Caring for the disabled elderly. Who will pay?* Washington, DC: The Brookings Institute.

Chapter 7

End-of-Life Care

Karen O. Kaplan

A dozen years ago, I stood at my mother's bedside in an intensive care unit. At 78, my mother was extremely frail and nearing death. She had suffered a massive coronary and was being kept alive by a respirator and multiple medications. She was no longer alert enough to know that I was there and was unable to talk to her doctors. However, it was clear that she was in significant pain. Her kidneys were failing and the doctors had requested permission to initiate dialysis. They awaited my "yes" or "no" decision.

CHANGES IN END-OF-LIFE CARE

Some of the history of the growing social movement to improve care and caring near the end of life tells us what led to the development of advance care planning and brought the difficult issue of the end of life back to living rooms and kitchen tables, doctors' offices and hospital rooms. A profound change occurred between the 1950s when death was treated as a normal part of the life cycle and people died in the arms of loved ones, in peace and with dignity, and the 1990s, when deaths like my mother's were the rule rather than the exception.

These five decades saw the production of modern medical miracles. The era of powerful antibiotics was born. Dialysis, transplant, and laser surgery were developed. Life support machinery and techniques became commonplace, as did diagnostic procedures that identified serious illness at its onset and tracked it throughout its course. Ecstatic at the marvels that were routinely brought about in doctors' offices and hospitals, the medical profession and the public began to view death as a failure—a failure of the medical profession to find the right intervention to stave off the death of the patient who was dying and yet not expected to get better.

As death became an increasingly repugnant enemy, it was moved further out of sight. Death became a taboo subject in homes and hospitals and, sadly, in medical schools. We taught our medical students and other health care professionals little if anything about using the increasingly superb technology to ease a dying person's symptoms or engaging in compassionate communication to ease spiritual pain and family suffering. And we taught the public practically nothing about exercising its right to determine what kind of care is received at the end of life.

Slightly more than a decade ago, a cultural revolution began—quietly, slowly—but tenaciously. A small group of visionary leaders embarked on multifaceted efforts to improve the care, and caring, that people receive as they near the end of their lives and took into consideration the needs of the families in this process. These efforts and the changes that accompanied them came about for many reasons, two of which were vitally important and highly visible.

One significant phenomenon prompting change was the shift of the media spotlight to issues concerning dying and death. The media extensively covered groundbreaking legal cases such as *Cruzan v. Director, Missouri Department of Health*[1] and *Washington v. Glucksberg* and *Vacco v. Quill*[2] and, by doing so, substantially raised public awareness of end-of-life issues.

The media also paid rapt attention to Kevorkian's "assisted suicides." Both careful and sensational reporting of Kevorkian's activity focused the nation's attention on two important facts: not everyone wanted to prolong the dying process with technologic interventions, and far too many people suffered needlessly atrocious deaths.

---

[1] *Cruzan v. Director, Missouri Department of Health*, 497 U.S. 261 (1990) recognized the individual's right to refuse unwanted treatment.

[2] *Washington v. Glucksberg et al.*, 177 U.S. 2258 (1977). *Vacco, Attorney General of New York et al. v. Quill et al.*, 117 U.S. 2293 (1977) recognized a state's right to make assisting in a suicide a criminal act.

The second event driving the emerging cultural revolution was the publication of a landmark study, SUPPORT (SUPPORT Principal Investigators, 1995). This study documented, for the first time, serious deficiencies in care for dying patients and their families. Its appearance in the professional and lay press and subsequent publications by the American Board of Internal Medicine, "Caring for the Dying" (ABIM, 1996), and the Institute of Medicine, "Approaching Death: Improving Care at the End of Life" (Field & Cassel, 1997), resulted in professional education initiatives and public engagement efforts. Collectively, these efforts are bringing about welcome changes in the way people die in America, among them increasing acknowledgment of palliative and hospice care and increasing acceptance and practice of advance care planning.

PALLIATIVE CARE

Discussion about life's ending is still not common. Far too many persons have little or no knowledge about the options available for quality end-of-life care. There is little public (and, as yet, too little professional) awareness of the components of a "good death."

However, knowledge and interest in palliative care is growing. Palliative care is defined as "the active total care of patients whose disease is not responsive to curative treatment." The goal of such care is to provide the best possible quality-of-life for patients near the end-of-life and their families (ABIM, 1996). "Palliative care:

- affirms life and regards dying as a normal process
- neither hastens nor postpones death
- provides relief from pain and other distressing symptoms
- integrates the psychological and spiritual aspects of patient care
- offers a support system to help patients live as actively as possible until death
- offers a support system to help the family cope during the patient's illness and in their own bereavement" (ABIM, 1996).

Treatment, even surgery, is part of palliative care when the benefits of the prescribed treatment in relieving symptoms outweigh any disadvantages.

To provide a baseline of knowledge, one of the most widely disseminated publications concerning end of life was developed by Last Acts, as part of a Robert Wood Johnson Foundation national campaign to improve care and caring near the end of life. This document, *The Precepts of Palliative Care* (Last Acts Task Force, 1997), is broadly considered by most experts as the gold standard for care near the end of life. A consumer version, *A Vision for Better Care at the End of Life: Five Principles of Palliative Care*, focuses attention on the uniqueness of each person's death. The five components comprising quality end-of-life care are:

1. Pain and other physical and psychological symptoms should be alleviated and comfort maximized by medical care that conforms to best-practice standards and is consistent with the person's values and preferences.
2. The physical and emotional environment should be as pleasant and supportive as possible and include time spent with loved ones and other people of choice.
3. Dying persons and their families should be cared for in a manner that respects inherent dignity.
4. Dying persons should be able to exercise personal autonomy (control) to the extent desired and feasible.
5. Dying persons should be able to explore issues of meaning and spirituality, with support from others as desired.

The hospice is a modality that offers palliative care and may be provided in the hospital setting or the home. Its philosophy and features are related to those in palliative care. Unlike the usual hospital setting, the hospice provides "palliative, rather than curative treatment; treats the person, not the disease; emphasizes quality, rather than length of life; considers the entire family, not just the patient; offers help and support to the patient and family on a 24-hour-a-day, seven-days-a-week basis" (Last Acts).

As palliative care and hospice programs continue to increase, persons at the end of life and their families gain a wider choice as to where and how they will live their last days.

ADVANCE CARE PLANNING

Advance care planning is the process an individual goes through to decide how he or she would like to live the last chapter of life—what medical treatments to seek, where to be, whom to be with, and how to complete life's business—the practical, emotional, and spiritual. As simple and straightforward as the name sounds, advance care planning is among the more emotionally and intellectually difficult tasks one ever faces.

Fortunately, there are now significant supports available to ease the advance care planning process. State and Federal advance directive statutes, although in some ways flawed, support and protect an individual's right to complete advance directives, including living wills and health care (medical) powers of attorney enforceable by law.[3] (See Appendix, p. 81) Myriad educational materials, in print and on websites, exist to guide people through the advance care planning process. Experts are beginning to be available to consult with and advise those making these important life—and death—decisions.

Experts[4] agree that there are three distinct stages of advance care planning, each of which has different characteristics and steps. The first step, often the most difficult to approach, involves "Planning Ahead" and encompasses the activities most commonly thought of as Advance Care Planning. The second stage, "Rethinking," occurs shortly after the onset of a serious illness that is likely to be life limiting, and the third, "Just in Time Revisions," takes place as the individual approaches death.

"Planning Ahead" is a gift to oneself and one's family. The last chapter of life is about living to the fullest extent possible. To do so requires rethinking and planning in advance about what matters most. The tasks one wishes to accomplish as life nears an end, (saying farewell, reconciliation, forgiveness, etc.), the ways in which one wishes to be treated by others (and the place one wants to be), and the balance of benefits and burdens associated with particular treatments are among the decisions to be considered. To help ensure that one's final weeks or months are spent in the desired way, in the preferred setting, and that family and friends understand and accept their roles in making it so, there are several steps that comprise Planning Ahead that should be completed at some time during adulthood.

1. *Sorting through values, needs, experiences, and wishes:* The experts say that if you've seen one death, you've seen one death. Just as every

[3]Living wills are statutory documents that permit individuals to delineate in writing the kinds of treatment they would or would not want when they near the end of life. Health care (medical) powers of attorney permit individuals to legally appoint someone (called an agent or proxy) to make medical decisions for them if they are unable to do so for themselves.
[4]For example, Joanne Lynn, Karen Orloff Kaplan, Mary Meyer, and Charles Sabatino.

person is unique, so too is each person's dying and death. To be certain that the dying process approximates one's wishes as closely as possible, it is essential that individuals contemplate those aspects that are most likely to be under their control. For example, is home or hospice or hospital the place to spend one's last days? And what about pain? Is complete comfort preferable to being fully alert and able to interact with family? What about aggressive and probably futile treatment such as resuscitation and artificial nutrition and hydration? Individuals' answers will reflect their life experiences and values and each person's answer will differ.

2. *Documenting preferences:* In situations in which an individual is unable to speak for him or herself, there are only a handful of ways in which that person's preferences can be determined. The most basic of these ways is a completed living will. A living will is used to document, with some specificity, one's treatment preferences, particularly concerning pain management, artificial nutrition and hydration, resuscitation, and place of death. Each state has different laws concerning the format and content of living wills, so locating a state-specific living will is crucial.[5] Making use of educational materials and available advice is a good way of ensuring that the completed living will is clear enough to cover most situations.

3. *Selecting an agent:* Every person facing death needs an advocate who will work with the health care providers and facilities to ensure that the person's preferences are known and implemented. Selecting an advocate (known as a health care agent or proxy) is one of the most important parts of Planning Ahead. The agent must be someone trusted, assertive, and fully knowledgeable about the patient and his or her preferences. The legal form that one uses to appoint an agent is called a *health care power of attorney* (or power of attorney for medical decisions). Again, states vary in their laws concerning the appointment process and content of the document. Thus a state-specific document is highly desirable.

4. *Talking, talking, talking:* Without the necessary conversations, the living will and health care power of attorney are simply pieces of paper. When needed, they may not be found. When available,

---

[5]*Last Acts Partnership* provides state-specific living wills and medical powers of attorney with complete instructions and a toll-free number for additional information and advice. The documents are free of charge through the organization's website: www.lastactspartnership.org; toll-free number is 1-800-989-WILL.

they may not be clear. When they are clear, various family members and/or the health care professionals may disagree. Once an individual completes a living will and appoints a health care agent, it is essential—indeed critical—that he or she talk with the agent, the doctor, and all family members likely to be at his or her bedside. Explaining the meaning of one's preferences, discussing various circumstances that might arise, and making sure that everyone understands and agrees is the best it can be, and death the best that it can be.

The second stage of advance care planning, "Rethinking," occurs when one receives a diagnosis of a serious, potentially life-limiting disease. It is hoped that the basic tasks associated with "Planning Ahead" have been completed much earlier. Now it is time to talk with one's doctors about the course of the illness, treatment alternatives, the associated benefits and burdens, and likely prognosis. In view of that information, are the decisions reflected in one's living will and the individual selected as one's agent still the right ones? If not, changes can be made easily. If one changes either a living will or appoints another agent, it is important to hold the conversations again.

Finally, as one moves closer to death, circumstances might lead to rethinking, once again, the decisions formerly made. As long as one is able to make decisions, "Just In Time Revisions" are possible and additional decisions, for example, about a "do not resuscitate" order, can be made.

Given the power of advance care planning directives for ensuring a "good death," it is surprising that more people do not complete them. Experts, such as Dr. Sean Morrison, suggest that only about 25 percent of the overall adult population in this country has completed advance directives. Even among individuals older than 65, the completion rate is just about 70 percent. Only when people are older than 85 does the rate of completing advance directives rise above 90 percent.

Today, the Baby Boomer generation is caring for many of those who will die in the coming years. By the year 2030, as many as 5.3 million Baby Boomers may be receiving long-term care and reaching the end of life (Kaplan & Byock, 2001). They should think and plan ahead for what they wish.

APPENDIX[6]

Partnership for Caring
Facts about Advance Directives

What are advance directives?
"Advance Directive" is a general term that refers to your oral and written instructions about your future medical care, in the event you become unable to speak for yourself. Each state regulates the use of advance directives differently. There are two types of advance directives: a living will and a medical power of attorney.

What is a living will?
A living will is a type of advance directive in which you put in writing your wishes about medical treatment should you be unable to communicate at the end of life. Your state law may define when the living will goes into effect, and may limit the treatments to which the living will applies. Your right to accept or refuse treatment is protected by constitutional and common law.

What is a medical power of attorney?
A medical power of attorney is a document that lets you appoint someone you trust to make decisions about your medical care if you cannot make those decisions yourself. This type of advance directive may also be called a "healthcare proxy" or "durable power of attorney for health care." The person you appoint through a medical power of attorney is authorized to speak for you anytime you are unable to make your own medical decisions, not only at the end of life.

Why do I need an advance directive?
Advance directives give you a voice in decisions about your medical care when you are unconscious or too ill to communicate. As long as you are able to express your own decisions your advance directives will not be used and you can accept or refuse any medical treatment. But if you become seriously ill, you may lose the ability to participate in decisions about your own treatment.

---

[6]Reproduced with permission of Partnership for Caring, Washington, DC. 1-800-989-9455; pfc@partnershipforcaring.org; http://www.partnershipforcaring.org

What laws govern the use of advance directives?
Both federal and state laws govern the use of advance directives. The federal law, the Patient Self-Determination Act, requires health care facilities that receive Medicaid and Medicare funds to inform patients of their rights to execute advance directives. All 50 states and the District of Columbia have laws recognizing the use of advance directives.

The booklet, "*Advance Directives and End-of-Life Decisions,*" available from Partnership for Caring, offers more information about advance directives.

REFERENCES

American Board of Internal Medicine. (1996). Caring for the dying. Identification and promotion of physician competency. Educational Resource Document, 215-243-1562.

Field, M. J., & Cassel, C. (Eds.). (1997). Committee on care at the end of life, Division of Health Care Services, Institute of Medicine. *Approaching death: Improving care at the end of life*. Washington, DC: National Academy Press.

Kaplan, K. O., & Byock, I. R. (2001). Living on the edge: Baby boomers face caregiving dilemma. In *Finding our way: Living with dying in America*. Coordinated by The Center for Advance Illness Care, VA Healthcare Network Upstate New York at Albany, Partnership for Caring and Last Acts (now Last Acts Partnership), Center for Death Education and Bioethics at the University of Wisconsin. Knight, Ridder/Tribune.

Last Acts Task Force on Palliative Care. (1997). The precepts of palliative care. Copies available at www.lastactspartnership.org

SUPPORT Principal Investigators. (1995). A controlled trial to improve care for seriously ill hospitalized patients: The study to understand prognoses and preferences of outcomes and risks of treatment (SUPPORT). *Journal of the American Medical Association, 274*, 1591–1598.

SUGGESTED READING

AARP. (2003, April). Beyond 50:03. A report to the nation on independent living and disability. AARP's Public Policy Institute.

Adelman, R. (2002, April 24). Presentation at Third Summit Meeting: *Can my eighties be like my fifties?* The New York Academy of Medicine, New York.

Arno, P., Levine, C., & Memmott, M. (1999). The economic value of informal caregiving. *Health Affairs, 18*(2) 182–188.

Cantor, M. H., & Brennan, M. (1993, September). *Growing older in New York City in the 1990s.* (Vol. 5: *Family and community support systems of older New Yorkers.*) New York: The New York Center for Policy on Aging of the New York Community Trust.

Center for Medicare Education. (2003). *Medicare and long-term care.* Washington, DC: *Issue Brief,* Vol. 4, No. 4.

Chen, Y. (2003). Funding long-term care: Applications of the trade-off principle in both public and private sectors. *Journal of Aging and Health, 15*(1), 15–44.

Kane, R. L. (1999). A new model of chronic care. *Generations, Integration of Care in a Changing Environment, XXIII*(2), 35–37.

Kayser-Jones, J., Schell, E., Lyons, W., Kris, A., Chan, J., & Beard, R. (2003). Factors that influence end-of-life care in nursing homes: The physical environment, inadequate staffing and lack of supervision. *Gerontologist, 43*(Special Issue II), 76–84.

Manton, K. G., & Gu, X. (2001). Changes in the prevalence of chronic disability in the United States black and nonblack population above age 65 from 1982 to 1999. *Proceedings of the National Academies of Sciences, 98*(11), 6354–6359.

McFalls, J., Jr. (2003). *Population Bulletin, 58*(4). (Electronic version). Population Reference Bureau. Retrieved 1/22/04 from www.prb.org/Template.cfm?Section=PRB&template=/ContentManagement/ContentDisplay.cfm&ContentID9789.

National Center for Health Statistics. (2003). As referenced on Population Reference Bureau website. Retrieved 1/22/04 from www.prb.org/Template.cfm?Section=PRB&template=/ContentManagement/ContentDisplay.cfm&ContentID9527

National Institutes of Health. (2003). *Report to Congress* (Electronic version). Retrieved 11/30/03 from http://aspe.hhs.gov/daltcp/reports/Hcwork.pdf

Noelker, L. S. (2001).The backbone of the long-term-care workforce. *Generations, Journal of the American Society on Aging, XXII*(1), 85–91.

Program offers new models for care of the elderly and disabled: $7M grant boosts Boston College Graduate School of Social Work study. (2004, January 22). *The Boston College Chronicle,* See also Robert Wood Johnson Foundation website, www.rwjf.org

Stone, R. I. (2000). Introduction: Consumer direction in long-term care. *Generations, Journal of the American Society on Aging, XXIV*(3), 5–9.

Stone, R. I. (2001). Research on frontline workers in long-term care. *Generations, Journal of the American Society on Aging, XXV*(1), 49–57.

U.S. Department of Labor. (2000). Balancing caregiving and work. Study commissioned by the U.S. House of Representatives.

Vladeck, B. (1998, June 16). *The future of long-term care.* Presentation at the Long-Term Care Planning Symposium, Mount Sinai Health Care Foundation, Cleveland, OH, pp. 3–4.

Vladeck, B. (2001, October 10). *Keynote address.* Presentation at First Summit Meeting: *Can my eighties be like my fifties?* The New York Academy of Medicine, New York.

Weiner, J. M., & Rivlin, A. M. (1988). *Caring for the disabled elderly. Who will pay?* Washington, DC: The Brookings Institute.

Chapter 8

Retirement, Lifestyles, and Roles: Leisure, Volunteering, and Work

OVERVIEW

Beginning in 2011, the Baby Boomers will begin reaching their 65th birthdays and soon thereafter will become eligible for retirement with full Social Security benefits. Even earlier, in 2008, these same Baby Boomers may, if they wish, opt for reduced SS benefits when they reach 62 years of age.

It is difficult to predict whether the Baby Boomers will maintain the latest trend toward delaying retirement. The Cornell Midcareer Paths and Passages Study, in 2000, found that the youngest Baby Boomers and the post-Baby Boomers anticipated retiring two years earlier than the leading edge of the Baby Boomers, who planned in 2000 to retire earlier than their parents' generation (Moen, Plassman, & Sweet, 2001). These expectations appear to be changing, perhaps due to the economic realities of recent years. Workers nearing retirement age are now reporting that they will continue to work because they cannot afford not to do so. Additionally, eight out of ten persons between the ages of 45 and 74 also say that they will continue working even if they are able financially to retire. John Rother (Rother, 2002) emphasizes that older workers today frequently do not have this choice.

Only a few years ago, the average retirement age had dropped to 57 but with the current economic uncertainty, older workers appear to be remaining in the workplace, if this is possible for them, and choosing to wait until their late sixties and beyond to retire. Eighteen million persons 55 and older are part of the labor force, and a recent AARP survey suggests that the numbers will grow (Duka & Nicholson, 2002). On the other hand, the current decline in the economy also means that older workers are vulnerable to downsizing and being forced into retirement. "For many workers, the traditional organizational career is rapidly becoming obsolete" (Moen, 1998) so that even without the current downturn in the economy, remaining in a job for lengthy periods of time is no longer the norm. Development of a global economy, technological change, a general shift to service economy, and concerns over productivity/competitiveness in the U.S. mean that the workplace is being restructured through downsizing and the disappearance of job ladders.

"Americans generally, and baby boomers in particular, are experiencing a disconnection between the traditional career path and the growing numbers of women in the workforce" (Moen, 1998). The career path, in the sense of moving up the ladder, is a male model, and women have always been "typically more constrained in the workforce" although, today, the notion of a career path is becoming outdated for both men and women. In the current economy and with the weakening career path, older workers nearing retirement age are at risk of losing their jobs to younger, less costly employees. Surprisingly, data compiled by the Labor Department's Bureau of Labor Statistics and reported in the *New York Times*, indicates that whereas younger workers have been hard hit by the current downturn in the economy, older workers, those over 55 years of age, appear to have escaped downsizing and layoffs. "Older people now make up 12% of the nation's workers, up from 10.2% in 2000." The increase in percentage is due to the thinning of the ranks of younger workers, but it also indicates that older workers have not lost ground during this recession, unlike their experiences during earlier downturns in the economy (Uchitelle, 2003).

WORK OR RETIREMENT?

Retirement is a relatively recent concept, a product of industrialization. Once self-employment, either on the land or as a craftsman, was replaced by working for a company employer, retirement came into being. It was further fueled both by the 1935 Social Security Act and by trade unions' advocacy for the right to leave the workplace with a pension, opening up positions for entering workers. Retirement today is viewed as a natural stage in the life cycle that is rightfully due to all in spite of Moen's warning that "the lock-step sequence of education, employment, and retirement is obsolete, a cultural relic of a society that no longer exists. What is required is a thoughtful reappraisal of existing life patterns" (Moen, 1998). Retirement as a stage in an individual's life, whether forced or a considered choice, spanned only a few years in the first half of the twentieth century. Today, with our increasing longevity, the retirement years may represent almost a third of our lives.

This expansion of the retirement years to a 25 to 30-year period places an economic burden on most persons. The role of work today, in terms of defining future income (pensions and Social Security) for retirement, is critical. To date, the Baby Boom generation has spent more than its parents' generation but has also saved less. Many Baby Boomers can expect to reach their retirement years with insufficient financial resources, and will be making hard choices between continuing in the work force or retiring. "Unless some fundamental policy changes are implemented, more Boomers will be spending their later years working just to make ends meet" (Simon-Rusinowitz, Wilson, Marks, Krach, & Welch, 1998).

Not everyone makes the decision to retire voluntarily. Approximately one third of the work force are forced into early retirement, often due to health reasons, and many of those who opt to retire at the age of 65 also make this choice unwillingly and out of necessity because of poor health. For those undriven by health factors, the choice between retiring and continuing to work increasingly depends on financial factors. The poor status of the U.S. economy today argues in favor of continuing work, as does the fact that there is no longer a penalty on earnings after the age of 65. It is still true that delaying receipt of Social Security until reaching the age of 70 results in higher Social Security benefits, but receiving full Social Security payments after 65 while still in the work force is no longer subject to deductions.

Choices to continue in the work force include working more years than anticipated, part-time work, consultant work, flextime, or participating in phased retirement programs that offer shorter hours/shorter work weeks or job sharing. Bickley Townsend speaks of phased retirement as "any arrangement that enables older workers to reduce their work hours and responsibilities for the purpose of easing into full retirement." In general, employers do not extend much flexibility to workers to enable this but the changing workplace and aging of the work force favor movement in this direction, and such practices may become more widespread (Townsend, 2001).

Even when in good health, not all Baby Boomers will have freedom to opt for work or retirement. For people of color and many women, the only valid question will be whether retirement is an affordable option (Stanford & Usita, 2002).

> Because these (white) men have historically enjoyed more generous pension benefits, they are better able to choose voluntarily whether to work longer or to retire. Working people of color, on the other hand, are more likely to be forced out of the labor market due to an inability to secure or maintain employment. Yet at the same time, they are also less well positioned to retire because of a lack of adequate savings or pension income. The financial fear often heard, "I can't work, but I can't retire either," captures the dilemma. [Hudson, 2002, p. 1]

We can expect to see a growing divide between the haves and the have nots, between the "pension elite" and low wage, non-pension workers. In addition, "younger Boomers may be more adversely affected by the pension decline than older Boomers; younger Boomers entered a tighter labor market and are likely to receive weaker benefit packages than their older counterparts" (Simon-Rusinowitz et al., 1998).

Nearly one half of workers retiring today work for pay at some point after retirement (Moen, Erickson, Agarwal, Fields, & Todd, 2002). Whether the Baby Boomers retire early, retire from one job to employment elsewhere, become part-time workers or consultants (what Moen refers to as "blurred" retirement), or remain longer in the work force, the majority will eventually experience full retirement. How will the Baby Boomers approach these retirement years? What are their expectations? How will they use their time during this life stage? Dr. Robert Butler, among others, suggests that there is a need to develop new social, political, and cultural roles for Baby Boomers in old age (Butler, 2001). There is a sense that the Baby Boomers will refashion retirement, just as they have done with every stage of their lives, but, as yet, there is no clear image as to what the result will be.

BABY BOOMERS' CONCERNS AND WISHES FOR RETIREMENT

Studies of today's retirees indicate that planning for retirement is positively related to better life quality in the retirement years. Planning is not only financial but includes health care needs, housing arrangements, developing hobbies/interests, and planning new careers. "For a large segment of society, retirement focuses on leisure, enhanced quality of life, and maintaining financial resources" (Stanford & Usita, 2002).

It is generally believed that the Baby Boom generation is failing to prepare financially for its retirement years or to contemplate the potential for poor health and the accompanying costs and caregiving needs. However, lack of preparation does not mean that there is lack of thought for the future. Baby Boomers' concerns for their retirement include questions about their income security related to the fear that they will have to work well into old age because they will be unable to afford to retire. Existing anxiety about current jobs and financial security may interfere with planning and saving for the future (Simon-Rusinowitz et al., 1998). Also of concern is the provision of care for their own parents, and a generalized anxiety about remaining independent. This anxiety does not, however, appear to result in planning for a potentially frail old age. Insurance companies offer long-term care plans to cover costs of possible nursing home and home care but these plans can be costly and there is no guarantee that they will be needed. Indeed, Baby Boomers are often unwilling to consider the possibility. Old age itself, whether accompanied by frailty or not, is viewed as an option to be rejected.

ANTI-AGING MEDICINE

The Baby Boomers' denial of the aging process and their concurrent enthusiasm for products and therapies that mask signs of aging or purport to delay or reverse physical manifestations of aging are troubling to many observers. An active and growing anti-aging movement appeals to the Baby Boom generation which grew up in a youth-oriented cultural period (Binstock, 2003). Ironically, this youth-centered period resulted from the existence of the large number of Baby Boomers themselves, and now that the leading edge of the cohort is reaching its late middle years, the youth-focused culture, instead of giving way to a celebration of positive aging, remains dominant.

Face lifts, hair transplants, tummy tucks, and other surgical interventions to keep the body looking youthful are no longer reserved for the rich and famous but are increasingly popular at earlier and earlier ages. Simultaneously, the Baby Boomers prove to be a large market for anti-aging products (skin creams, potions, herbal remedies, etc.) and therapies (enema regimes, magnetic contraptions, live-cell injections, exercise programs, etc.). Use of anti-aging products, especially dietary supplements, increased after the Dietary Supplement Health and Education Act of 1994, which relaxed federal regulation of these products.

A year earlier, in 1993, the American Academy of Anti-Aging Medicine (A4M) was founded. The organization claims a large membership of scientists, health professionals, and physicians throughout the world and via conferences, publications, and its website, promotes anti-aging medicine and its message of the extension of the life span. The growth of this anti-aging movement is met with concern by the traditional scientific and medical communities, which view the anti-aging movement as a "fraud and purely money-making business" (Binstock, 2003).

There has long been friction related to competition for research funding between researchers of age-related diseases and the biogerontologists, with the biogerontologists receiving less recognition but arguing that it is preferable to focus on the mechanisms of the aging process as these are the underlying risk factors for all age-associated disease. In spite of their differences, both factions are currently united in their opposition to the anti-aging movement. A 2001 workshop, convened to answer the question "Is there an anti-aging medicine?" determined that "in spite of considerable hype to the contrary, there is no convincing evidence that currently existing so-called 'antiaging' remedies, promoted by a variety of companies and other organizations, can slow aging and increase longevity in humans" (Butler et al., 2002). The National Institute on Aging discredits anti-aging claims for pills containing antioxidants, DNA, and RNA, as well as for dehydroepiandrostene (DHEA) and growth hormones and urges consumers to use caution in use of anti-aging hormones (NIA, 2002). The U.S. General Accounting Office goes even further, stating "anti-aging products pose potential for physical and economic harm" (USGAO, 2001). Recently, over 50 researchers in the field of aging collaborated to inform the public of the distinction between the "pseudoscience" antiaging industry and the genuine science of aging (Olshansky, Hayflick, & Carnes, 2002).

The human life span has been extended through medical interventions, improved nutrition, and a decrease in disease-related behaviors. There is also evidence that certain medical interventions delay or prevent disease, such as drug treatments to prevent peptic ulcers/stomach cancer; lipid-lowering drugs for those with high LDL cholesterol, and antihypertensive agents for high blood pressure, as do behavioral practices of regular exercise and use of high fiber in diets, sun-blocking products, seat belts, and avoidance of tobacco (Butler et al., 2002). These interventions and practices have extended life expectancy but it is calculated that even if we were eventually able to eliminate cancer, heart disease, and stroke, life expectancy would only be raised another ten years into the upper nineties (Olshansky, Carnes, & Cassel, 1990). This is very different from the extension of life to 150 years and beyond heralded by the anti-aging movement. In the future, cell replacement therapy may be helpful in reversing some adverse effects of aging and allowing us more years in good health but this, also, is not expected to increase our life expectancy (Butler, 2001). In fact, there is no evidence that any product can slow the aging process in humans although there is some encouraging research that suggests a restricted caloric intake does slow the aging process in animals. A diet for humans that requires eating 30 to 50% less than normal and that is begun early in life may be the solution for someone wishing to live to 140 or more years (International Longevity Center, 2001). The individual who wishes to practice this regime must be prepared to be always cold, and always hungry, and it seems clear that very few would have the determination and stamina to adhere to such a regimen.

Enthusiasm of Baby Boomers for anti-aging products and therapies is fueled by a desire to remain healthy and outsmart the aging process but generally succeeds only in maintaining a lucrative industry. In contrast, the workshop convened to examine anti-aging medicine faults society for not practicing healthy habits. The U.S. population is failing "to take advantage of our genetic potential for longevity by engaging in practices which lead to premature onset of the degenerative diseases associated with aging" (ILC, 2001). Fifty percent of the U.S. population is considered obese, our diets are poor, and only 15% of those over 65 years of age exercise regularly. If the Baby Boomers, as well as Americans of all other ages, could change these behaviors, it is predicted that life expectancy would increase by another ten years (ILC).

LIFESTYLES

In spite of insufficient financial planning by many Baby Boomers and an unwillingness to envisage themselves as being frail in old age, with need for long-term care and its accompanying costs, it appears that, on the whole, Baby Boomers are giving thought to their post-retirement lifestyles. There is considerable variation in the degree to which individuals plan for lifestyle changes after retirement, but it appears that volunteering, belonging to social clubs, pursuit of hobbies, self-development through sports and physical exercise, travel, and education are all areas that interest Baby Boomers and feature in their hopes for the future (Moen et al., 2001).

Participants at the summit meetings spent some time discussing and defining their wished-for ideal retirement. There was general agreement that, whatever their individual differences, Baby Boomers wish to spend their retirement years as members of intergenerational neighborhoods in which the older persons' activities and interests are fully integrated into the life of a self-directed, supportive community. There will be opportunities for spiritual and personal growth through volunteering, education, and travel. The Baby Boomers, who reached young adulthood in the '60s, wish to be useful in a social role, contributing to the community, and to have easy access to programs and services. Their twin desires for their old age are to maintain their independence and to have one or more persons to talk to, to be connected to others. Freedom to be independent and freedom to take advantage of all opportunities are valued.

SOCIAL ISOLATION

Retirees are vulnerable to social isolation without the ongoing contacts with others that the workplace provides. The majority of today's retirees enter their retirement years as healthy, active, and independent and any social isolation that occurs is through individual choice and preference. However, as we age, loss of spouse or partner and the advent of chronic age-related disease become more likely. Those who live alone and are in poor health may become increasingly isolated from their community, family, and friends. Those without family members nearby—the never married, childless, or those who live at a distance from family—are especially at risk. Studies show that caregivers at a distance (adult children, nieces, nephews, and siblings) tend to have emotionally close and caring relationships equal to caregivers who live close to their older family members even though the regular face-to-face contact is missing. With modern technology bringing us video and audio phone and Internet connections, family members and friends can maintain high quality social contact with each other even over long distances, thus mitigating against social isolation. Baby Boomers and their families will benefit from this emerging technology to a greater degree than their parents and grandparents generations, today's elderly population.

Modern technology notwithstanding, there is concern that a significant number of Baby Boomers, aging into their late eighties and nineties in poor health, will experience social isolation with all its potential physical and psychological downsides—malnutrition, confusion, loss of contact with reality, and increasing poor health. New and expanded support programs, both formal and informal in structure, need to be developed and integrated into the life of each community to help minimize these outcomes.

Today, it is the senior centers, social clubs, religious organizations, and volunteer groups that help to keep older persons who live alone connected to the larger community. Baby Boomers appear not to be members of fraternal and service clubs to the same extent as their parents and grandparents, nor do they express overwhelming interest in joining senior centers after retirement. This trend suggests that avenues for social contacts enjoyed by the current older population may not exist for the Baby Boomers. New and innovative programs and gathering points are needed to fill this void. Existing efforts to reach out to the elderly homebound also need to be expanded and reconfigured. This might be accomplished through building links between health and social services and the community at the local level to ensure that no one becomes socially isolated unless it is by choice.

Avoidance of social isolation as an objective of government has implications for public transportation and housing. Rural elderly may experience social isolation, even when not in chronic poor health or confined indoors, if they have no means of transportation. They require available and accessible means of moving within and outside their local communities, as well as do suburban and city dwellers. Some of the projected living arrangements and housing for the Baby Boomers in their older years are designed to eliminate lonely and isolated old age. This ought to become a consideration in all housing planning at every level, as well as a factor to be considered by individual Baby Boomers as they prepare for a future old age.

INCREASED LEISURE TIME: WHAT TO DO?

With the increasing life expectancy, the nature of retirement in the U.S. is already changing. For the first time in history, retirement is viewed as a period of life in which to pursue interests, to travel, and to acquire new skills and knowledge. Regardless of the financial concerns overshadowing retirement plans, it is anticipated that the Baby Boomers, in large numbers, will continue to view retirement from this perspective as a period of life in which to enjoy themselves. In fact, studies indicate that "most Baby Boomers who are getting close to retirement are looking forward to having fun, more so than any preceding generation" (Moschis, 2002).

Marketing to the senior population is a big business, and the imminent arrival on the retirement scene of the Baby Boomers is creating business opportunities in the travel, hotel, sports, and hospitality industries, catering to all levels of disposable income. Baby Boomers are likely to be barraged with options to take up a new sport, participate in adventure holidays, discover untapped artistic talents, take a cruise, and so forth, and have the option to choose from a range of activities and interests. For those with low incomes, there are discounted weekend getaways, trailer parks, community centers, and public recreational activities.

Similar marketing, though at a less strident level, is aimed at the desire to use retirement years to learn. Higher education institutions invite senior students into the classrooms and offer summer sessions and continuing education in a variety of topics. Educational organizations are likely to offer even more opportunities in the years ahead as the value of the senior market is recognized as a source of additional income. The current popularity of the Elderhostel educational vacations and tours is a further testament to the older population's interest in learning. The Baby Boomers are expected to continue in this tradition. An educational model, practiced in many European countries, is the Third Age movement, which is low cost and draws upon the knowledge and skills of older persons. The model operates at the local, community level, with older persons leading classes for their peers in a variety of subjects. It is a model that could be easily replicated in the United States.

Senior centers, the core of the Administration on Aging's services to older persons, offer meals, socialization, cultural programs, classes, and access to services such as transportation and benefits. Currently, the senior centers are locked in a struggle to remake their image, with the objective of continuing to provide services and a community activity center for an aging, increasingly frail population while also meeting the socialization and learning needs of the well, independent, young retirees. Baby Boomers rarely envisage senior centers as featuring in their older years but, at the same time, they speak of the desire to be part of supportive communities. This is a role for which the senior centers are designed. Accordingly, the centers are reshaping themselves by adding intergenerational programs, health and fitness centers, political action groups, and so on to attract new participants from today's young retirees and to position themselves to meet the interests and needs of the future older population.

VOLUNTEERISM

Baby Boomers are viewed as a vast potential social resource for the U.S. (Freedman, 2002). Large numbers of older persons in our country's future will prove enormously beneficial, as it is anticipated that a significant proportion of these older persons will offer their time to service, health, religious, cultural, and business organizations of all kinds. A volunteer's hours of service contribute not only to society but to the individual volunteer's sense of being useful, one of the wishes for retirement expressed by the Baby Boomers.

Many of today's older persons have chosen to become volunteers. A national organization, the Senior Corps, includes three volunteer programs for persons over the age of 55 years. These are the Foster Grandparents, the Senior Companions, and the Retired Service Volunteer Program (RSVP). The Senior Corps has over 2 million older persons volunteering their time and skills for an average of four hours each week. It is probable that an equally large number of older persons volunteer under the aegis of other organizations, such as Volunteers of America and Literacy Volunteers, or volunteer independently on an individual basis. The Baby Boomers intend to continue this tradition of volunteer service and, given their stated desires and increased years of good health, may well contribute to a greater degree than does the current older population.

The Baby Boomers also foresee that part of their initial retirement years will be devoted to caring for frail parents entering their late eighties and nineties and perhaps, also, for grandchildren, enabling parents to remain in the work force. The Baby Boomers are not averse to taking on family care but do express a wish that formal services, with professional knowledge and skills, will be available to share the responsibilities of any long-term care that is needed. Volunteer assistance might also be forthcoming, given the numbers of Baby Boomers that are expected to be interested in volunteer activities.

SUCCESSFUL AGING

There is considerable interest, now that our old age spans 20 to 30 years, in what constitutes successful aging and how each individual can aspire to become successful in the process. Certainly those Baby Boomers who acknowledge the fact of their aging must be as interested in the concept as their parents' generation.

Research findings over the past half century suggest that what many once viewed as signs of normal aging are, in fact, the effects of disease, albeit age-related disease such as Alzheimer's disease, arthritis, or vascular problems. Thus, successful agers are those who avoid age-related disease and reach old age without the accompanying deficiencies. Rowe and Kahn (1998) proposed this definition of successful aging in the late 1980s and, with the award of a McDonnell Foundation grant, undertook a study and further defined successful aging (or aging well) as freedom from disease and disease-related disabilities, high cognitive and physical functioning, and continuing engagement in life. This definition has its detractors, who argue that it consigns most older persons to be judged as aging unsuccessfully even though older persons, when asked to rate themselves subjectively, overwhelmingly classify themselves as successful. Alternative definitions suggest that successful aging is doing the best with what one has (Baltes & Carstensen, 1996) or that it includes older persons experiencing chronic, age-related conditions with minimal resulting cognitive and physical disabilities (Strawbridge, Wallhagen, & Cohen, 2002).

Whatever definition seems the most appropriate, the lesson to be drawn from the debate is that although we may not be able to manage our genetic makeup, each of us can take steps earlier in life to increase the possibility of aging successfully. Exercise, a healthy diet, avoidance of smoking, and an interest in life, which translates into participation and friends, all make the avoidance of physical and mental disease more likely and increase our chances that we will enter old age as independent and contributing members of society.

REFERENCES

Baltes, M. M., & Carstensen, L. L. (1996). The process of successful aging. *Ageing and Society, 16*, 397–422.

Binstock, R. H. (2003). The war on anti-aging medicine. *Gerontologist, 43(1)*, 4–14.

Butler, R. N. (2001, October 10). Seven deadly issues. Keynote address at Summit Meeting: *Can my eighties be like my fifties?* The New York Academy of Medicine, New York.

Butler, R. N., Fossel, M., Haman, M., Heward, C., Olshansky, J., & Perls, T. (2002, September). Is there an antiaging medicine? *Journal of Gerontology Series A: Biological and Medical Sciences, 57*(9), B333–B338.

Duka, W., & Nicholson, T. (2002, December). Retirees rocking old roles. *AARP Bulletin,* 3.

Freedman, M. (2002). Civic windfall? Realizing the promise in an aging America. *Generations: Retirement: New Chapters in American Life, 26*(11), 86–89.

Hudson, R. (2002, Spring). People of color and the challenge of retirement security: Inequities cast a shadow. *Public Policy and Aging Research Brief,* 1.

International Longevity Center. (2001). Is there an "anti-aging" medicine? An interdisciplinary workshop of the International Longevity Center-USA. New York.

Moen, P. (1998). Recasting careers: Changing reference groups, risks, and realities. *Generations: The Baby Boom at Midlife and Beyond, 22*(1), 40–45.

Moen, P., Erickson, W., Agarwal, M., Fields, V., & Todd, L. (2002). *The Cornell retirement and well-being study: Final report.* Ithaca, NY: Cornell University. 2000.

Moen, P., Plassmann, V., & Sweet, S. (2001). The Cornell midcareer paths and passages study: Summary. Ithaca, NY: Cornell University.

Moschis, G. (2002). Retirement and retirees: An emerging business opportunity. *Generations: Retirement: New Chapters in American Life, 26*(11), 61–65.

National Institute on Aging. (2002). Life-extension. Science or science fiction? Website http://www.nia.gov/health/agepages/lifeext.htm

Olshansky, J., Hayflick, L., & Carnes, B. (2002, August). Position statement on human aging. *Journal of Gerontology, Series A: Biological and Medical Sciences, 57*(8), B292–B297.

Olshansky, S. J., Carnes, B. A., & Cassel, C. (1990). In search of Methuselah: Estimating the upper limits to human longevity. *Science, 250,* 634–640.

Rother, J. (2002). Presentation at third Summit Meeting: Can ny eighties be like my fifties? 10/5/02. The New York Academy of Medicine, New York.

Rowe, J., & Kahn, R. (1998). *Successful aging.* New York: Random House (Pantheon).

Simon-Rusinowitz, L., Wilson, L., Marks, L., Krach, C., & Welch, C. (1998). Future work and retirement needs: Policy experts and baby boomers express their views. *Generations: The Baby Boom at Midlife and Beyond, 22*(1), 34–39.

Stanford, E. P., & Usita, P. M. (2002). Retirement: Who is at risk? *Generations: Retirement: New Chapters in American Life, 26*(11), 45–48.

Strawbridge, W., Wallhagen, M., & Cohen, R. (2002). Successful aging and well-being: Self-rated compared with Rowe and Kahn. *The Gerontologist, 42*(6), 727–733.

Townsend, B. (2001, Spring). Phased retirement: From promise to practice. *Issue Brief.* Cornell Employment and Family Careers Institute, 2(2).

Uchitelle, L. (2003, September 8). Older workers are thriving despite recent hard times. *The New York Times,* National Section, pp. A1, A15.

U.S. General Accounting Office. (2001). *Health products for seniors.* (Publication No. GAO-01-1129). Washington, DC: U.S. Government Printing Office.

Chapter 9

Living Arrangements

INTRODUCTION

Closely intertwined with health status and income security for Baby Boomers is the subject of housing. As they have done at each stage of their lives, Baby Boomers are likely to have a significant impact on the kind and form of housing they create to meet their needs both as they enter old age as active, productive members of society and as they age over the following twenty years, perhaps to become frail and in need of assistance. Baby Boomers need to reinvent retirement in the activities and interests that they pursue and in terms of where they live and what living arrangements they favor.

CURRENT LIVING ARRANGEMENTS AND OLD AGE

Current housing and living arrangements are already diverse, and it is anticipated that many of the changes we are witnessing in the living arrangements of older persons are likely to continue. The 2000 census indicated that 55% of non-institutionalized older persons, representing 41% of older women and 73% of older men, live with their spouse. Due to lower life expectancies for men, the percentage of women living with a spouse decreases with age so that by the age of 75 only about 29% of women live with a spouse (Administration on Aging, 2002).

Almost one third of non-institutionalized older persons live alone. This translates into 40% of older women and 17% of older men. Not surprisingly, as these statistics show, the proportion of older persons living alone increases with advancing age. Almost half of women over 75 years of age live alone. These statistics are of some concern to gerontologists suggesting that, with the growing older population of the Baby Boom generation, future years will experience large numbers of old persons living alone. However, this may not necessarily be a problem as individuals of the Baby Boom generation are more practiced at living alone than their parents' and grandparents' generations. The increase in the never married, divorce rates, and later marriages means that many Baby Boomers may have known earlier life phases of living alone, suggesting that, for those in good health, the experience of living alone in old age may be less difficult than it is for today's 75+ newly widowed women.

The remaining 10% of non-institutionalized men and 19% of women live with other persons, either family or friends. This includes the traditional family makeup of an elderly parent living in the home of an adult child as well as non-traditional structures. For instance, in recent years, there has been an increase in grandparents raising grandchildren, two generations of the old living in one home, and older parents caring for developmentally disabled adult children. In the past this latter population had a short life expectancy. This is no longer true. Persons with developmental disabilities now enjoy an average life expectancy, living into their sixties and beyond, but still requiring care from their 80 and 90 year old parents (Prosper, Sherman, & Howe, 2000).

The 2002 census found that in 80% of households headed by older persons the dwellings were self-owned, with a full 73% of that group owning their homes free and clear. The remaining 27% were renters. This relatively-high ownership of homes may be due not only to older houseowners having paid off their mortgages but also to the practice of middle-income couples downsizing at retirement and relocating, using proceeds from the sale of the family house to buy outright. The median year of construction of homes occupied by older householders is 1963, as compared to 1970 as the median age of construction for all householders (AOA, 2002). This is an important statistic. Housing is a significant factor in health outcomes for disabled elders. The ability of individuals to live as independently as possible is often dependent upon the characteristics and construction of the homes in which they live. "Research suggests that a 'user-friendly' home not only increases its safety and usability by the disabled resident but may also facilitate the efficient delivery of in-home care" (Newman, 2003, p. 106). A 1995

American housing survey (U.S. Census Bureau) found that 14% of the older population had a "housing-related disability," that is, a disability due to the housing environment, such as inability to navigate steps leading in and out of the home.

LIVING IN THE COMMUNITY

The preferred option for the current older population and also of the Baby Boomers is to remain in the community during their older years. Today's elderly and their families only consider institutional living as a last resort if the older person needs round-the-clock or custodial care and there are no family members available or capable of providing the necessary assistance. It is unlikely that this preference will change. It is common knowledge that the majority of frail older persons "do better" at home among their own familiar community and possessions where they are able to continue their daily activities and retain some measure of independence. Apart from this benefit, less public funding is required to care for individuals in the community, leading to the current public policy that favors the provision of services in the home environment over institutionalization.

There are a variety of options available to today's older population. These are expected to remain and possibly increase in the years ahead.

Remaining in the Original Home

A substantial number of older persons remain in their homes. The increasing popularity of reverse mortgages enables homeowners on fixed incomes to afford the costs of staying in place. Although low-income renters are unable to utilize this financing method, they may be fortunate enough to be in rent-controlled or rent-stabilized apartments and/or eligible for protection from rent increases through a Senior Citizen's Rent Increase Exemption (SCRIE) program.

NORCs

The tendency for older persons to remain in place results in a phenome-non known as Naturally Occurring Retirement Communities (NORCs), that is, communities in which there are clusters of older persons who have "aged-in." In recent years there has been a growing interest in providing needed services for older residents in defined NORCs, especially in areas of low income. The growing number of assessment and service delivery projects in these communities may well serve as a model for community-based integration of services for older persons in the future. NORCs are addressed in greater detail in the following chapter.

Downsizing: The Move after Retirement

Most Baby Boomers, once retired, will stay in place, at least initially. The future will see an increase in all kinds of areas occupied by older Americans and will include older persons opting to stay in their own homes as well as those who select a specific area as a desirable place to live for older persons (Golant, 2002). A move from the home in which the children were reared to a smaller, less costly home may be the choice for many. This move may coincide with a relocation to a more manageable climate, a lower cost of living, or a move closer to family members. Traditionally, the warmer states, especially Florida and Arizona, have been viewed as the favored retirement locations. This is now changing, with preference being given to areas that have lower costs of living. As of 1990, the top states welcoming the most older persons included New Jersey, Washington, Virginia, and Georgia (Longino, 1995). In the last decade, the areas with the fastest growing populations of those over 65 were small and medium cities in the South and West in states other than Florida and Arizona (Golant). Some move to areas that offer easily accessible amenities, such as New York City, which is now attracting the return of older suburbanites who value the cultural and recreational activities and ease of access to them.

A recent study of home buyers 50 years and older by the National Association of Home Builders found that the majority of buyers are not cashing out the equity from the family home and downsizing into a smaller, less costly home or apartment but are paying more for a home for their retirement years with, often, the latest amenities such as structured wiring, pull-down shelves, and low-maintenance housing materials (America's Seniors, 2003). Meanwhile those remaining in their own homes are using the equity they have built up in paying for high-tech options and universal design features. It seems that the older wave of Baby Boomers is not only looking to utilize the latest technological offerings but is also planning for a future that includes potential frailty, seeking renovations that include wheelchair accessible rooms and well-positioned electrical outlets, handrails, ramps, and so forth. Others are building an Elder's Cottage on the grounds of their homes or remodeling to incorporate self-contained units within their homes for use by older parents. It is reported that the demand for in-law or mother/daughter suites has been increasing in new home developments in Florida, with as many as a third of all homes in one new development including such a suite (Koprowski, 2002).

Retirement Communities

A small percentage of our future elderly will "radically change their residential milieus" and move into "active adult retirement communities" (Golant, 2002). These communities are designed for the "young," active, independent older person. They offer spas, recreational facilities such as golf courses and tennis courts, and a planned community of low-maintenance, owner-occupied units (houses or apartments). Residents under the age of 50 are generally not allowed and children are permitted only as visiting guests. These communities offer a lifestyle geared to leisure pursuits and, as such, are not readily affordable to most. In recent years, newer retirement communities have become even more luxurious and are appealing to the well-to-do.

Shared-living Residences

There is growing interest in the establishment of informal cooperative groups. Small groups (5 to 6 older persons) of friends plan and participate in shared living arrangements, either pooling resources to purchase a home together or moving into the home of one of the group. Glorified by the TV sitcom, "The Golden Girls," this appears to be of interest to many Baby Boomers, who view it as a way of maintaining full independence while enjoying shared costs and companionship. The theory is that whereas generally the participants are independent and active at the outset, if frailty arises, the group members will care for each other and be mutually sustaining. There are too few such arrangements in place, and those that do exist are not yet "old" enough for there to be any definitive findings on the viability and worth of this modality. It may fall to the Baby Boomers to venture into this area in large enough numbers to enable society to judge its utility and effectiveness.

Independent Senior Housing

A less expensive form of the retirement community, independent senior housing, has often been developed with the assistance of government funding and/or the sale of bonds by religious groups, fraternities, or local government. Such retirement communities are designed to provide homes in areas that lack appropriate and affordable housing for seniors. Few additional services and amenities are offered and residents must be able to live independently or make their own arrangements for needed assistance.

Rent Subsidies

Under the terms of federal housing legislation, a proportion of public housing is available for low-income persons over the age of 62. Rent subsidies are awarded. Subsidized rent may also be available in non-public housing for persons 62 or older with an income 80% or less of the median income in the specific area. Currently, 11.2% of all subsidized housing units are occupied by disabled individuals over 62—approximately 520,000 persons (Newman, 2003). Unfortunately, these rental assistance programs are limited and unable to meet the requests of all those who are eligible. Housing stock for older persons with low income is lacking throughout the United States and there is little promise that this situation will improve in the near future.

Home Care and Community Services

Whether Baby Boomers remain in their own homes or elect to enter retirement communities, senior housing, or shared living arrangements, home care and community services will be needed to enable those who become frail to remain within their communities. Current policy in favor of care in the community is promoting a growing variety of programs delivering different levels of home care including visiting nurse services, home attendants, home aides, companion services provided by private agencies, not-for-profit groups, and paid or volunteer care providers. Medicare only covers a limited number of home care hours after hospitalization. For those who are income eligible, Medicaid covers home care costs with the number of covered hours dependent on each individual state's provisions. For those older persons whose income is above Medicaid eligibility and who are ineligible or have exhausted the Medicare-covered services, the cost of private home care can be prohibitive.

A second drawback to care provided in the community at home is that it is frequently disconnected from the larger health care system. Medical centers and health care systems are beginning to enter the home care arena but this is not universal, and one of the enduring difficulties is the fragmentation of health services. Individuals are too frequently discharged from the hospital without needed home care in place or, never having been hospitalized, are unable to secure appropriate home care that could help them avoid future hospitalization. In addition, home care workers are generally underpaid, undertrained, and undersupervised, contributing to uneven standards of care. Coordination and increased quality of care are two areas in which the Baby Boomers can have an impact through advocacy and involvement in the planning of home health care at the Federal, state, and community levels.

Technology

Equally as important as services is technology in enabling older persons to remain in the community. We are already seeing the role advancing technology can play, and with the Baby Boomers offering a sizable market for technological inventions and assistive devices, this is clearly an area that will grow in importance. Technical advances in universal design allow the home environment to be user-friendly for older persons (ramps, non-slip floors, low maintenance building materials, etc.) and in the outside environment, technology is playing a major role in increasing mobility. Lightweight folding chairs, electric carts, and mobile scooters are allowing individuals who otherwise might be confined indoors to move freely and efficiently within their communities.

INSTITUTIONAL LIVING

Institutional living for the older person first brings to mind nursing home care. Today, however, the nursing facility is only one among a variety of institutional living formats that are becoming available. The increasing numbers of older persons living long lives with chronic health problems, and the specter of even greater numbers in the future, with the Baby Boomers adding to the senior market, are leading to a growing emphasis on other forms of institutional living to fill the gap between independent living in the community and full nursing facility care.

Assisted Living

Today, assistive or assisted living is a generic term covering any integration of housing and supportive services or assistance. "Assisted living is a form of residential long-term care that combines services and housing for individuals who are unable to live independently. Undefined by statute or regulation at the federal level, assisted living is essentially a new and expanded term for residential care settings that have existed for many years" (Center for Medical Advocacy, 2003). This type of living arrangement is constantly changing. Consumer demand, investors, and those public regulations that do exist continue to reshape the assisted living sphere. At the same time the involvement of health and insurance companies, frequent business mergers, and partnerships between developers and hotel chains or universities all contribute to fluctuations in the assisted living market (Prosper et al., 2000). Consumers want the option of housing plus social and health services when they are needed, whereas the developers are still seeking the most appropriate mix that will prove economically viable over time.

An early attempt to fill the gap between independent community living and full nursing home care was known as congregate housing, in which older persons rented their own self-contained living units with the opportunity to participate in congregate meals and various social and recreational activities. This model was not universally successful, partly because promoters overestimated the demand and underestimated the level of care that was needed. However, congregate housing became the forerunner of assisted living as individual entrepreneurs joined continuing care retirement communities and the larger nursing homes in expanding their continuum of care, resulting in "assistive living facilities providing a non-invasive support system in a residential setting" (Zimmerman et al., 2003).

Assisted living is the fastest growing form of senior housing in the United States. In spite of overconstruction, which led to a cutback in the early 1990s in some locations, new assisted living facilities are opening every day. A 1998 survey conducted by the assisted living industry found that assisted living accounted for 75% of new senior housing (Tinsley, Ronal, 1998). The Assisted Living Federation of America represents over 6,000 for-profit and not-for-profit providers and, as of 2003, it is estimated that 20,500 assisted living properties exist with a total of 2.27 million apartments among them. A recent survey ascertained that half of all those living in assisted living facilities are over the age of 85 (Hawes & Phillips, 2000).

There are basically three general models of assisted living. At one end of the spectrum are small facilities grouping up to ten persons together. These facilities may be known under a variety of names—personal care homes, homes for adults, domiciliary care, adult foster care, sheltered housing, or senior group homes. Shared bedrooms, bathrooms, and living space are the norm. These facilities may or may not be regulated in any way.

The second model is housing that generally accommodates more than ten persons. Housing with services is marketed to older persons who are already in need of some support—meals, supervision of drug regimens, transportation, social activities, and so forth, but do not require nursing home care. Adult homes, which have existed for many years, are included under this category. They are designed for older persons who are unable to live alone but do not require extensive medical care. The homes provide meals, transportation, housekeeping, personal care and 24-hour supervision and may be licensed under state regulations.

The third modality is the life care or continuing care community which offers independent housing for active, healthy retirees with the promise of continuing care, enabling residents to move into more sheltered housing with support services as needed and, eventually, if required, to obtain full nursing home care, all on the same campus. Such communities have high initial buy-in costs and carry high monthly service charges against potential future use of the more intensive care services and are therefore, by necessity, costly and out of the range of the average older person's financial resources.

The absence of any overarching federal regulations and differing state regulations result in a wide range in cost, quality, and actual deliverables in assisted living programs. Whereas uniform regulations and licensing are needed to ensure quality care, proponents of such legislation stress the importance of flexibility to enable a wide range of assisted living modalities in all price ranges to coexist.

Nursing Facilities

Only about 4.5% of the older population, about 1.56 million persons, reside in a nursing home. Although this is a small percentage, the likelihood of entering a nursing home rises with increasing age, with over 18% of those over the age of 85 living in such a facility. The horror of being warehoused in a nursing home is inextricably mixed with the public's ideas of old age but in fact, nursing home care today is mostly reserved for those individuals of all ages who require round-the-clock nursing care that cannot be provided at home in the community.

The cost of nursing home care is high. Medicare covers a short stay and is designed for purposes of rehabilitation after hospitalization and eventual return to living in the community. For those who are eligible, Medicaid will assume the costs once Medicare coverage is exhausted. For those who are not Medicaid eligible, the costs of nursing home care can quickly deplete resources and may reduce income to the point that Medicaid eligibility occurs. Currently, insurance companies are promoting policies to cover the costs of potential nursing home care. These programs are relatively new and undersubscribed so that the fees are high. Once an increased number of persons buy into the programs, it is anticipated that the insurance premiums will decrease.

PREPARING FOR THE FUTURE

There is a wealth of housing options for older persons designed to meet the needs of the active, healthy older person as well as to cater to the frailer individual requiring social and health services. However, many of these options are neither affordable nor accessible to all. Baby Boomers are adamant about their desire to remain at home in the community setting even if they become frail and require support. A Cornell University study of late-midlife workers and retirees found that this population expects to age in place but their expectations of living in highly supportive environments are uniformly low (Robison & Moen, 2000). If the Baby Boomers' dream is to be realized, an increase in senior housing of all kinds is necessary, and a system of well-coordinated home health care and community services, as part of the continuum of overall care, is required. According to Dr. Donna Shalala, "Housing needs imagination," and Nicolas Retsinas, director of the Joint Center for Housing Studies at Harvard University, says, "This healthier and wealthier generation (of Baby Boomers) will redefine senior housing" (Schutz, 2002).

Housing developers are targeting Baby Boomers with special amenities. The AARP and National Association of Home Builders, which may be self-motivated, advise Baby Boomers to consider remodeling their homes sooner rather than later if they plan to stay and age in place. Universal design homes that are gero-friendly are the ideal. At the same time, efforts are needed by health and social service providers as well as the Baby Boomers, the future consumers, to put in place coordinated support services and to utilize technology to find new ways of keeping individuals in the community while maintaining mobility and independence.

ANTICIPATING THE FUTURE: MARIE AND MARCOS

Baby Boomers, participating in the first summit meeting, looked into the future and identified the ideal living arrangements and lifestyle they wish for themselves when they reach the age of eighty. This is Marie and Marcos on their 80th birthdays in 2026.

Marie

Marie lives in a housing development that is both architecturally and environmentally age friendly. It includes a variety of housing options. She lives in a one-bedroom ground floor apartment in a three-story building and is friendly with several of her neighbors who live in her building and in the townhouses on the other side of the communal garden. Marie's married daughter lives across town and they see each other fairly frequently and chat on the phone. Marie cooks for herself as well as eating out at the nearby coffee shop two or three times a week with her sister or one or more of her friends.

Marie moved to the apartment ten years ago. When her husband died she sold their family home and purchased the apartment with the proceeds. The remaining monies, plus her social security, pension, and income from a few investments, allow her to live fairly comfortably although she watches her finances carefully. She is planning to live to be 100.

Marie has easy access to social, educational, and recreational programs. She attends the Thursday book group and is a member of a political action group at the Community Center, although she participates more for the social aspects than from any real desire to change the world. She has registered for an Italian conversation course at the Community College, where she also uses its recreational facilities, swimming twice a week.

Marie was a kindergarten teacher for many years and she now helps out for a couple of hours each weekday at the Children's Learning Center. Sometimes she answers the phone or assists with mailings to the parents but mostly she is in the classroom with the little ones, reading stories and providing hugs as needed.

Marie's health care is covered by Medicare and she attends the local health care center where she has access to a group of three persons—a nurse, a physician, and a social worker—all of whom know her well. She sees the nurse on a regular basis to have her blood pressure checked and will see the doctor if there are any medical problems. When she fell last winter and was homebound for a few days, the doctor visited her at home while the social worker arranged for an aide to come daily to help her with bathing and to prepare meals. Marie knows that if she becomes frail and is unable to care for herself, she will be able to get the help she needs from the health center and will be able to remain in her home.

Marcos

Marcos lives in a trailer on the edge of town with his second wife, who is also 80 years old. When they first moved there, the trailer was situated among fields but now the town has grown outwards and surrounds them. Marcos was a farm worker for most of his working life and his second wife worked in the school cafeteria. They are both in good health and are able to "live off" their monthly Social Security checks and a small inheritance that Marcos received from his uncle. Seven of the eight children they have between them and several of the grandchildren live upstate but they all talk on the phone and the entire family gets together for all the holidays. Their youngest child is 53 years old and lives nearby. They visit her about once a week.

Marcos knows everyone and goes downtown almost every day to hang out with his friends in the Court Square in the summer or, when the weather is bad, at the community recreational center. He is also active in several organizations and is a deacon at his church. Marcos does not drive a car but there is bus transportation right outside his door that can take him to most of the places he wants to go.

His wife accompanies him once or twice a week when she meets her friends or when it is one of her volunteer days at the hospital. Marcos was recently invited to speak to a class at the local college about life in the town when it was a farming community. He was a big hit with the students and has already been invited to speak to other classes. He jokes about starting a new career as an inspirational speaker.

Marcos and his wife see a doctor once a year for checkups. When they were first married, Marcos used to worry about what would happen if one of them or their teenage children got really sick, as they could not afford to pay medical bills. Happily, there is now a community health clinic in town to which they belong. The center provides the annual checkups and advises on preventive care and the doctors will visit patients in their homes if necessary. Dental care is also available. The costs of their health care are fully covered by Medicaid.

Marcos and his wife plan to live and die in their trailer and have refused all suggestions to move upstate and live with one of their children. Marcos keeps the home in good repair. His nature is to worry, and he used to wonder about what his wife would do if he dies first because he knows she will be unable to keep the trailer in good condition. But their church now has a volunteer group that helps out with repairs, and the social service office at the community center promises to find whatever help is needed to enable people to stay in their homes, so Marcos knows all will be well.

Marie and Marcos are living the kind of lives that today's Baby Boomers wish for their future. They are lives of independence, secure income, and good health, connected to supportive networks of family and friends with the freedom and ability to choose among a variety of cultural, creative, spiritual, recreational, educational, and travel opportunities. Firmly entrenched government programs, providing income support, housing, and health care, are readily accessible to those in need.

THE REAL FUTURE

In reality, Baby Boomers are likely to experience technological benefits that will change lifestyles in ways we can barely foresee. At the very least, Marie will be participating in her Italian conversation class online from within her home, and her volunteer work at the child center will include responsibility for instant messaging to parents and use of a nutrition monitor to record the children's nutritional needs. Marcos might remain at home also, instead of traveling downtown to hang out with his friends, by using a video/audio chat room. Closed circuit monitors will be installed in the homes of older persons to enable constant monitoring. Individuals will be able to use the technology to record blood pressure, temperature, and other vital signs and have the results immediately placed in their personal health data file. At the sign of any deviation from the norm, health care professionals will be alerted. Similarly any fall or need for assistance will be recorded and the necessary help dispatched within seconds. Communicator microchips will provide immediate auditory and visual contact with anyone on the user's personal call list. If solitude is desired, the older person can make use of an individual home entertainment center, installed on the wrist, to gain access to any music, movie, book, or artwork ever created.

These and other technological advances may or may not become commonplace. In any case, we can plan for the lifestyles that we desire in our futures by strengthening the organizations and structures that we already know. The following chapter on naturally occurring retirement communities offers a model to do just that.

REFERENCES

Administration on Aging. (2002). *A profile of older Americans: 2002 living arrangements.* http://www.aoa.gov/prof/Statistics/profile/4.asp

America's Seniors. (2003, August). *Baby Boomers, seniors continue 'buying-up'; new study to reveal preferred home features, financing trends.* Retrieved August 27, 2003, from http://www.todaysseniorsnetwork.com/boomers'_housing.htm

Center for Medical Advocacy, Inc. (2003). Medicare and assisted living. *Health Care Rights Review, 4*(1). Washington, DC: Author.

Golant, S. M. (2002). Deciding where to live: The emerging residential settlement patterns of retired Americans. *Generations, Retirement: New Chapters in American Life, 26*(11), 66–73.

Hawes, C., & Phillips, C. (2000, February). *High service or high privacy assisted living facilities, their residents and staff: Results from a national survey.* National Study of Assisted Living Facilities, U.S. Department of Health and Human Services. Report available at: http://aspe.hhs.gov/daltcp/reports/hshp.htm

Koprowski, G. (2002, July 20). Add-ons for new live-ins. *The Washington Post.* As cited by Minnesota Planning in Minnesota Issue World. (2002,November). http://www.mnplan.stats.mn.us/issues/scan.htm

Longino, C., & Fox, R. (1995). Retirement migration in America: An analysis of the size, trends, and economic impact of the country's newest growth industry. Houston: Vacation Publishers.

Newman, S. (2003). The living conditions of elderly Americans. *Gerontologist, 43*(1), 99–109.

Prosper, V., Sherman, S., & Howe, J. (2000). Living arrangements for older New Yorkers. In *Project 2015. The future of aging in New York State. Articles and briefs for discussion* (pp. 35–41). Albany, NY: New York State Office for the Aging.

Robison, J., & Moen, P. (2000). A life-course perspective on housing expectations and shifts in late midlife. *Research on Aging, 22*(5), 499–532.

Schutz, L. (2002, November). Baby Boomers redefine senior housing. Minnesota Department of Administration website. http://server.admin.state.mn.us

Tinsley, R. (August, 1998). 1998 ALFA Survey highlights—Assisted Living Federation of America. Nursing Homes.

U.S. Census Bureau. (1995). American Housing survey 1995. Washington, DC: Department of Housing and Urban Development.

Zimmerman, S., Gruber-Baldini, A., Sloane, P., Eckert, K., Hebel, R., Morgan, L., et al. (2003). Assisted living and nursing homes: Apples and oranges? *Gerontologist, 43*(Special Issue II), 107–117.

Chapter 10

Aging in Place: Shaping Communities for Tomorrow's Baby Boomers—Naturally Occurring Retirement Communities (NORCs)

Fredda Vladeck

As America's Baby Boomers approach retirement age, there has been much worry and speculation about the impact on society. The focus of this speculation has been directed toward Social Security and Medicare, but while this discussion of the burdens of caring for deficits-driven, dependent old people has been occurring, another discussion has been quietly taking place across the country, focused on transforming communities into good places in which to grow old. Where and how retired Baby Boomers are going to live is a question central to the future shape of our society and to the economic impact of aging.

The overwhelming majority of seniors (89%) are staying put, preferring to remain in the homes they have lived in for years. This preference has been steady over almost twenty years, despite a proliferation of age-segregated communities and purpose-built senior housing. Currently, only 4.5% of seniors reside in nursing homes and only 7% live in age-segregated housing such as retirement villages, subsidized senior housing, assisted living facilities, and continuing care retirement communities (CCRCs). Although some segment of the older population will always desire or need purpose-built housing, even the retirement of the Baby Boomers will not change these proportions any time soon. As AARP reported in *These Four Walls . . . Americans 45+ Talk about Home and Community*, more than four out of five people surveyed intend to remain in their current homes with 82% of them preferring to receive services at home rather than moving if they need help in caring for themselves (Greenwald & Associates, 2003).

The "graying of America" is happening in communities large and small, from dense urban neighborhoods and developments to sprawling suburbs and remote rural towns. As the numbers continue to grow, older people will constitute increasingly larger percentages of the residents in many of our neighborhoods and communities. *Naturally occurring retirement communities* (NORCs), identified in the early 1980s by Michael E. Hunt (Hunt & Hunt, 1986), a professor of architecture and urban planning at the University of Wisconsin, is the term used to describe neighborhoods and housing developments originally built for young families in which a significant number of people are now 60 years old or older. Although Hunt originally used this term to describe a cluster of buildings in Madison that had experienced a large in-migration of people nearing retirement, most NORCs evolve over a period of years as those who moved in as young adults age in place. The older residents in NORCs are an increasingly heterogeneous population, healthier than ever before, living with less disabling chronic conditions, and possessing a wide range of interests, talents, and expertise. In many of these communities the older residents were the pioneers who built the schools, playgrounds, and other institutions that made these communities good places in which to raise young families. Few, if any, comparable roles or natural gathering places now exist for older people in the communities they originally helped build.

We are gradually understanding that communities play a critical role in how well people age. According to Richard M. Suzman, Associate Director of the Behavioral and Social Research Program at the National Institute on Aging (NIA), "community and neighborhood are important. So is the level of positive integration, neighborliness, looking out for others . . . which is . . . associated with higher life expectancy and better life" (Kilborn, 2003, p. A22).

Good places to grow old are characterized by opportunities

- to provide avenues for older people to take on positive roles (versus the stereotype of old people as a mass of needs);
- to empower older people and promote civic engagement (versus people who are acted upon);
- to promote social connectedness and a reweaving of the social fabric as earlier connections fray (versus home care policies that keep older people locked behind their front doors); and
- to develop an array of flexible and calibrated supports as needs arise (versus providing services one hip fracture at a time).

As Baby Boomers and communities age, the mechanisms and policies to ensure that communities can support "successful aging" as well as respond to changes in individual needs over time need to be developed. They will not emerge spontaneously.

A NEW MODEL EMERGES

Over the last twenty years, New York has led the way in developing a promising new model in response to the aging-in phenomenon occurring in many of its high-rise apartment buildings and dense communities. Called NORC-Supportive Service Programs (NORC-SSPs), these are collaborative financial and programmatic partnerships between housing entities, the residents, health and social service providers, government, and philanthropy to organize and locate a range of coordinated health care and social services and group activities on site in the housing complexes. Together, these partners assess the needs, interests, and resources in a community and design a program that will promote independence and healthy aging by engaging seniors before a crisis and responding with flexible, resident-specific services as needs oscillate. Eligibility for services and participation in activities is based on age and residence rather than on functional deficits or economic status. The existing categorical and entitlement programs (Medicare, Medicaid, and services under the Older Americans Act) are some of the important tools that are utilized in response to specific situations but, contrary to most service delivery models, they are not the only ones. Additional supports and services are developed to pick up where the public programs leave off to find ways to reintegrate seniors into the life of their community once an acute episode has subsided, and to support seniors in actively managing and maintaining their health.

The prototype of the NORC-SSP model was developed in 1986 in a large, ten-building, moderate-income cooperative in the middle of Manhattan (Penn South Mutual Redevelopment Houses). Built in 1962, many of Penn South's original 6,200 residents were trying to remain active and busy, dreading the day when a fall or serious health problem might limit their ability to participate in community life. It also had its share of problems, with confused residents wandering, losing keys, and forgetting to pay their monthly maintenance charge. Working with this author, who was a social worker at a local hospital, the resident Board of Directors conducted a survey to determine the needs of its frailer residents and the aspirations of all its residents as they aged in place. This process led to the creation of the Penn South Program for Seniors, which was funded initially by philanthropy. Within several years, the program exceeded expectations and the housing company became a financial partner, allocating funds from its operating budget for program support. The success of this model led to its replication in two other communities in 1992.

In 1995, New York State passed legislation creating the NORC Supportive Services Program Initiative with $1 million (increased to $1.2 million in 1996) granted annually to promote the development of 14 programs. Twelve are located in New York City. This was a pioneering effort by a state to create policy that would change how services for seniors are defined and organized, where they are delivered and to whom, and how they are financed. The legislation established thresholds for the extent of the senior population needed to achieve economies of scale in service delivery, defined the geographic boundaries of a naturally occurring retirement community, and established an ownership interest in a program through a public-private financing formula that required a housing company's financial participation. In 1999, the city allocated another $4 million annually to this effort, which resulted in additional grants to the existing 12 state-supported programs and the development of 16 new programs. Modeled after the state legislation, the city legislation modified some of the definitions to reflect the density and close proximity of large housing developments and to increase the government role of financing in these pubic-private partnerships (see Table 10.1).

There are now 27 NORC Supportive Service Programs in four of New York City's five boroughs. Almost 46,000 seniors live in a mix of

TABLE 10.1 NORC-SSP Coalitions for Participation: New York State and New York City

| | Population Threshold | Type of Housing Development | Geographic Boundaries | Sources of Required Financial Support | | | Additional Sources of Support |
				Government	Housing Development	Other Required Support	
New York State	50% of units with heads of household 60 years old or older or Minimum of 2,500 heads of household 60 years old or older.	Built with government assistance for moderate- and low-income families (rentals, cooperatives, and public housing)	Housing development with one or more building under a single management structure	50% or up to $150,000 annually per program. Ranges from $50,000 to $143,000	Minimum 25% cash match from housing company. Public housing is exempt.	25% cash or in-kind contributions of dedicated staff time for health care providers) and/or philanthropic support	In-kind contribution of space Client fees for group activities Legislative grants Resident directed fund raising Grants from local businesses Targeted philanthropic grants

(continued)

115

TABLE 10.1 (*continued*)

	Population Threshold	Type of Housing Development	Geographic Boundaries	Sources of Required Financial Support			
				Government	Housing Development	Other Required Support	Additional Sources of Support
New York City	45% heads of household 60 years old or older and minimum count of 250 or Minimum of 500 heads of household 60 years or older	Built for moderate- and low-income families (rentals, cooperatives, and public housing)	Single or multiple housing developments within a 1/4 square mile radius	Two-thirds, or up to $200,000 annually per program. Ranges from $45,000 to $200,000	Minimum 1/6 of DFTA grant cash match required from housing company. Public housing is exempt	Minimum of 1/6 of DFTA grant match required: philanthropy and/or contributed dedicated staff line (usually from health care provider)	Same as above

Source: United Hospital Fund Aging in Place Initiative "A Good Place to Grow Old." Fredda Vladeck

age-integrated developments. Programs range in size from a single building with 275 of its more than 500 residents over the age of 60, to a sprawling 12,000-unit complex in which 4,300 of its 30,000 residents are seniors. Two programs are in two-story garden apartment complexes, with the remaining 25 located in high-rise apartment developments. Seventeen programs are located in moderate income cooperatives in which the residents have an ownership interest, seven are in the public housing developments of the New York City Housing Authority, and four are in privately owned developments (2 rental and 2 cooperative) for moderate and low income individuals.

New York City's NORC-SSPs are financed through a combination of public and private sources. Government dollars (state and city) leverage matching funds from the participating housing entities (public housing is exempt) and philanthropy; other sources of support are local fundraising and membership fees for activities, as well as in-kind supports from the health care partners and the housing companies. Operating budgets range from $148,000 to more than $700,000.

NORC-SSP SERVICES

The structure of a NORC-SSP is predicated on the axiom that the sum is greater than its parts. It brings the diverse partners together to create a shared mission and vision of the program, establish a governance structure (including resident representatives) with accountability to the whole, and set forth the range of activities and services to be delivered. A lead agency (in most instances the social service provider) coordinates the work of the partners and provides the day-to-day management at each site.

Staffed by social workers and nurses, the NORC-SSP service design framework integrates four core elements:

- **Social work services** include information and referral; benefits and entitlements advocacy; assistance negotiating the systems and services available from the wider community; biopsychosocial assessment and support through casework, case management, service coordination, and monitoring for changing status of clinically complex or fragile individuals; and education and support for clients, paid and unpaid caregivers, and family members.
- **Health care related services** include individual care management to help seniors live with and manage chronic conditions and ad-

dress acute situations; the provision of non-reimbursable but necessary monitoring, care coordination, and support to maintain frail individuals at home; physical assessments, regular blood pressure monitoring and individual instruction; advocacy in negotiating the myriad health care systems; coordination with the primary care physicians and the on-site social workers; and health promotion, prevention, and wellness programs.

- **Educational and recreational opportunities** are diverse and designed to engage the broadest mix of seniors living in a community. Lectures on a wide range of topics, an array of classes, discussion groups, support groups, health chats with health care professionals are all provided. The list is limitless and is often defined by the seniors themselves. Although managed and organized by the professional staff, many of the classes and activities are identified and led by the seniors.
- **Volunteer opportunities** make it possible for seniors to take on new roles in their communities as program ambassadors, leaders, and program extenders in addition to those of consumers of service. Volunteer knowledge and understanding of their communities are instrumental in informing the planning process during a program's formative stages; setting program priorities as programs evolve; and identifying the resources, talents, and skills within each community. There are over 800 resident volunteers in New York City's NORC-SSPs, performing more than 42 different kinds of functions ranging from the individual support services (reader of mail, mender of clothes, translator, escorter, friendly visitor, and the like); to the provision of programmatic activities (discussion leader, teacher, peer insurance counselor, etc.); to the provision of administrative and development support (fund raiser, librarian, receptionist, event coordinator, writer and designer of marketing and communication materials, and statistician for community needs assessments).

Often additional services need to be developed to respond to the specific characteristics or needs of each community. Because programs do not have a narrowly prescribed set of services that they must deliver, they have the flexibility to customize their offerings to reflect community needs. Depending on its unique community characteristics, a program may need to develop transportation services in car-dominated or remote areas of the city, daily money-management assistance in those communities in which many seniors have little or no family close by, on-site gero-psychiatry services in a significantly aged-in community, or subsidized emergency home care for a community with limited resources for and access to in-home services.

LESSONS LEARNED

Based on such a large number of programs and close to 20 years of programmatic experience, it is clear that successful development of a NORC-SSP requires working in different ways and doing things differently. Historical service delivery models are increasingly rigid and bureaucratic, attempting to fit people into neat service boxes based on functional deficits as a way to ration fewer and fewer resources. They are the antithesis of the new paradigm of service delivery, and do not fit well with its inherent flexibility, responsiveness, and person-centeredness.

What is needed to develop this new model of service delivery?

1. **One size does not fit all**. Each community is unique, and so programs cannot be cookie-cut. The first step in developing an on-site supportive program is an assessment of a community and its residents to understand the community context in which seniors live and the resources available within them. Without a process that identifies a community's strengths, potential resources, concerns, goals, and aspirations, service providers run the risk of doing no more than locating on-site to react to crisis situations. Each community is made up of distinct population groups, each with its own history, culture, formal and informal social structures and sources of support, and ways of communicating.

2. **Roles are maintained throughout the ages**. Seniors need to be involved across the program spectrum, beginning with the planning and design of a new program and then participating as appropriate in the provision of services and in functions that help sustain and maintain the program. This approach is rooted in a strength-based approach to aging that empowers seniors to become actors and leaders in their community rather than individuals who are acted upon.

3. **Engagement is for everyone**. Programs must maximize the potential to engage seniors at all functional levels and abilities before a crisis occurs. Having a connection before a crisis increases the

likelihood that if and when help is needed, there is a trusted professional to whom one can turn, rather than a stranger who primarily
sees the deficits, however temporary they may be.

4. **Can you hear me now? It's about connections**. Opportunities
need to be created for seniors to connect to one another and to a
NORC-SSP or other supportive program in a variety of ways and for
a variety of reasons. The way most seniors get connected to services
in this country today is as a result of crisis. If a program is primarily
targeted to individuals with functional deficits, economies of scale
may be achieved by locating services closer to the intended client,
but such a model does nothing to de-stigmatize the need for help
or reweave the social fabric by encouraging residents to identify and
take advantage of the richness a community has to offer.

5. **We need to move from parallel play in the sandbox to har-
monic convergence**. Building a partnership made up of diverse
groups and organizations takes time and a willingness on the part
of each partner to work toward a common goal. This is not easy—and,
depending upon the particular partner, may be impossible—to do.
Each has its own institutional mission, organizational language, culture of service, and operational style that influence the partnership
dynamic. It requires skilled leadership to help the partners reach
consensus on a shared mission; the delineation of the roles and
responsibilities based on the resources and expertise each partner
brings to the group; accountability to the partnership, not just to a
distant main office; and the way in which success will be understood.

6. **Power to the people**. Professionals must be willing to share
power with the very individuals they are trying to help. In this kind
of model, the helping relationship takes on a new dimension. Empowerment and facilitation to maximize the social capital of the residents
in a community are as important as concrete services based on a
solid clinical assessment, but require not only different skills but a
different attitude that treats them as partners not clients.

LOOKING TOWARD THE FUTURE

Over the past 18 years, the quality of life for many of New York City's
NORCs and the thousands of residents who live in them has been
transformed. From a single program in 1986 to 27 NORC-SSPs today,
New York City's population and housing environment has been a fruitful

arena in which to develop and test a new service delivery model based on the paradigm grounded in our richer understanding of the tasks of aging and the needs of older people. As these programs continue to evolve and mature, there is much work still to be done to apply this model to naturally occurring retirement communities in other types of environments.

There are many questions that need to be answered if this model is to extend more broadly to communities less dense and more spread out than the apartment buildings of New York City. Efforts are already underway to modify the urban-dense model of New York City to fit the spread-out, single family homeownership communities found in less dense urban areas as well as suburban communities. Several philanthropic organizations are supporting activity in two suburban-like communities in New York (northeastern Queens and Plainview-Old Bethpage on Long Island) to identify appropriate organizational structures and capacities on which to build SSPs in the absence of unitary housing corporations. As a matter of public policy, New York City's NORC-SSP model stands out for its scope, the number of different projects involved with a single model, and the extent and duration of support from state and local governments. At the federal level, under earmark appropriations enacted by Congress in 2001 and 2003, the U.S. Administration on Aging has made grants to Jewish Federations in 14 cities to develop NORC-SSPs. Some of these cities are adapting the New York City model to their specific community characteristics. Others are struggling first to define their communities' geographic boundaries and target populations before tackling the issue of what services to provide.

Although government's involvement in the conversation about how to make our communities more livable for seniors is important, there is much activity happening outside government's purview. From the Partners for a Livable Community in Maryland to the nationwide AdvantAge survey project designed to understand the extent to which communities are elder-friendly, clearly this is a subject matter and area of interest whose time has come. Perhaps the most heartening thing is the extent to which seniors are taking matters into their own hands. In many parts of the country, they are not waiting for government or professionals to act. Almost every day, this author hears from or about a group at work on organizing its community. We have much to learn from these efforts as the older generation harnesses its lifetime of skills, knowledge, and experience, and transforms its communities into good places in which to grow old.

REFERENCES

Greenwald, M., & Associates. (2003). *These four walls . . . Americans 45+ talk about home and community.* Washington, DC: AARP.

Hunt, M. E., & Hunt, G. G. (1986). Naturally occurring retirement communities. *Journal of Housing for the Elderly, 3*(3/4), 3–21.

Kilborn, P. T. (2003, July 31). North Dakota town's payoff for hard lives is long life. *The New York Times,* p. A22.

Vladeck, F. (2004). *A good place to grow old: New York's model for NORC-supportive service programs.* New York: United Hospital Fund.

SUGGESTED READING

Freedman, M. (1999). *Prime time: How baby boomers will revolutionize retirement and transform America.* New York: Public Affairs.

Rowe, J. W., & Kahn, R. L. (1998). *Successful aging.* New York: Pantheon.

Chapter 11

Health Care Professionals and Their Education

Geriatrics is a comparatively new field for medicine and the other health care professions (e.g., nursing, social work). What is known and practiced today in meeting the health care needs of older persons is still evolving. Delivery of health care for older persons in the future may well be very different than it is now. This will be partly because of the greater numbers of older persons seeking health care and the shift away from institutions to the community for those requiring long-term care. In addition, the Baby Boom generation has different expectations from those of their parents and these will shape the nature of health care as the Baby Boomers enter their older years.

Delivery of today's health care adheres to a medical model. It is geared to responding to acute care needs with an emphasis on managing symptoms and effecting cures. In spite of the growth in health maintenance organizations, the involvement of health insurance companies, and their combined impact on what and when health care is provided, fragmentation of services and a general lack of coordination is evident. An older person with one or more chronic health conditions is likely to be receiving care from several medical specialists, all of whom are treating a single health condition, generally without reference to each other's care plans. A continuum of care from hospital to nursing home to community or vice versa is slowly emerging as health care systems and medical centers seek to provide care at all levels. However, this is not yet universal and too many of today's elderly patients are discharged from acute care before links to needed care in the community are established, or else they are unnecessarily admitted to institutional care for lack of community-based care. Meanwhile preventive care, while acknowledged as preferred and cost effective, is rare.

The Baby Boomers are asking for complete control over all aspects of their lives and deaths, and tend to be alert to their own health, aware of every nuance, and, if insured, quick to seek medical care. Use of alternative and complementary treatments is also popular (AARP, 2002). Although a growing consumer movement in health and long-term care is generally supported by policy makers, insurers, and health care professionals, health care professionals are concerned about consumer use of inaccurate or misleading information distributed in the media and on the Internet (Koop, 2003). Baby Boomers hope that aging will be different when they become 65, 75, 85, and 95, and are resolved that they do not want to grow old the way they see their grandparents and parents growing old. Health care professionals, health insurers, and managed health care systems need to rethink how health care will be delivered (Mezey, 2002).

Dr. Mathy Mezey describes how she envisages health care of the future, drawing upon the personal experience of a family member in need of cardiac surgery. In searching for the best care, the family was directed to the Family Centered Care offered at the University of Michigan, which takes into account the relationship of the patients and their families/significant others to the health care system. The Center treated the patient within the family context and attention was given to the family's concerns and needs. Treatment with this holistic approach was excellent, and the many members of the extended family, who were in attendance as advocates to assure appropriate care, found that they were not needed in this role. The care was good, independent of the advocacy skills of several family members who are themselves health care professionals.

This experience is very different from the kind of health care that most older adults can expect to receive today. A frail 85-year-old woman, perhaps with some cognitive decline, must have health-knowledgeable family or friends to accompany her to medical appointments in order to provide the translation between her needs and the health care professionals that she will encounter. Today, our system requires bolstering by enormous numbers of people to assure that the care is good and relevant (Mezey, 2002).

The family-centered social health care model projects the kind of health care that Baby Boomers want for their future: a holistic approach that views the older person within the parameters of a family and community structure and focuses on total needs—medical, social, psychological, and environmental—in establishing care plans and delivering services. They want a social health care approach in which the patient/older person and family/friends are equal partners in decision making and provision of care. This is the approach that Dr. Ronald Adelman (2002) refers to as the "patient-centered model" of interaction, as opposed to the generally paternalistic approach existing today.

THE INTERDISCIPLINARY TEAM APPROACH

The holistic approach, if not the patient-centered model, is beginning to be recognized in today's preparation of geriatricians. Viewing and responding to the older patient's needs from the perspectives of overlapping systems—biological, psychological, social, dietary, and so forth—requires the knowledge and skills of a multitude of professional disciplines. Hence there has been increasing interest in interdisciplinary teamwork within the health care of older persons.

The National Institutes of Health held a Consensus Development Conference in 1987 and developed a strong statement in favor of interdisciplinary teamwork/collaboration as the most effective means of assessing and treating older persons with health problems (Solomon et al., 1988). This interest in interdisciplinary collaboration has been advanced in recent years in a mandate for the Health Related Services Administration (HRSA)-funded Geriatric Education Centers and the rationale for the Geriatric Interdisciplinary Team Training (GITT) Programs funded by the John A. Hartford Foundation.

Appropriate health care of older persons is viewed as multidimensional and best provided by a core team representing medicine, nursing, and social work, with other disciplines participating dependent on the patient's needs (e.g., physical therapy, psychology, nutrition, etc.). Rationale for the team approach is based on the reality that most older persons, with chronic health conditions requiring long-term care, present with a multitude of issues and needs that all need addressing. These may be medical, psychosocial, financial, and/or environmental needs that no one health care professional is equipped to address alone. The expertise and knowledge base of three or more different disciplines may be required (Solomon et al., 1988). Furthermore, the proposed treatments and interventions must be integrated as the older person's needs are dependent upon each other and cannot be dealt with in isolation. For instance, a physician may prescribe a drug regimen for a diabetic 83-year-old woman with high blood pressure and depression, but if the patient lives alone and is incapable of administering her own medications or shopping for herself, no benefit will be gained. The coordinated interventions of a nurse and social worker, focusing with the physician on the patient's overall needs, are necessary for a good out-come.

The team approach, although promoted by national leadership and influential foundations, represents a departure from the traditional methods of managing health care. The reimbursement system for care fosters fragmentation as it does not currently cover direct care by essential health care professionals (other than medical) and thus is not conducive to interdisciplinary care. In some settings, the individual contributions of health care professionals to patients, other than by physicians and nurses, are unrecognized for purposes of specific service reimbursement. As long as the medical model of care persists, an interdisciplinary model will remain elusive. A change in professional culture, in particular that of medicine and medical education, which would endorse a pattern of holistic integrated health care, is required if interdisciplinary care is to become the norm.

EMERGENT TRENDS IN HEALTH CARE DELIVERY

The field of geriatrics has evolved in response to the health care needs of older persons but these needs have not been highlighted in the education of professionals who are providing the care. Learning more about the needs of older persons and recognizing that "new directions in health and mental health care delivery have increasingly complicated the ability of individuals and families to navigate health care systems" (Volland, Berkman, Stein, & Vaghy, 2000), and that at the same time these new directions have placed new demands on social workers in health care, the New York Academy of Medicine undertook a two-year study. The purpose of the study was to identify the gap between social work education and current practice and to determine the skills needed by social workers dealing with the health and social care needs of an aging population. The study noted the following trends in health care that may have led to the present disconnect between training and practice.

- shift from acute care to chronic illness and diseases of aging
- increased emphasis on market forces and cost control
- emphasis on measuring outcomes of health care interventions
- increased recognition of social and environmental determinants of diseases
- increasing roles of families, broadly defined, in provision of home care
- increased patient participation in health care decisions (Volland et al., 2000).

Educators of health care professionals need to acknowledge these trends and adjust professional training as needed. For instance, health care professionals are involved in long-term management of chronic disease; are shifting their practice focus to ambulatory, outpatient settings; are encouraging disease prevention and health promotion; and are improving overall health status by offering interventions for specific populations (Volland et al., 2000).

The acute inpatient care of the individual still requires attention, but knowledge and skills need to be developed to enable health care professionals in all disciplines to "fit" their practice to the changes we are experiencing. What we are learning about today's elderly in practice is gradually being introduced into education, but as the Baby Boomers age, there will be new knowledge to absorb and the current trends in health care can be expected to continue and become even more pronounced. At the same time that the professional schools are adjusting their curricula to reflect the changes, they are faced with the need to attract more individuals into the field of geriatrics.

CURRENT STATUS AND LACK OF PROFESSIONALS

There is an overall shortage of health care professionals in all disciplines. The shortage is particularly acute within the nursing profession—126,000 hospital nursing positions are currently unfilled (Jacoby, 2003). For the older population, the shortage is further exacerbated by the fact that very few of the health care force have received specialist training/education in caring for older persons. This is so even though the majority of hospitalized patients are over the age of 65. Geriatrics among the medical profession has long been ignored in favor of specialties such as cardiology and pediatrics and the same is true within the other disciplines.

NURSING EDUCATION

There are approximately 2.2 million practicing Registered Nurses in the country. Ninety percent of them are women. The average age of nurses is 47, which means that many of them are members of the Baby Boom generation themselves and are juggling family, work, and parent care. Most of these 2.2 million nurses have had no formal preparation in geriatrics, neither as students in their basic preparation program nor since then in terms of continuing education. A recent study found that only about 23% of undergraduate nursing programs include a required course in geriatrics. This contrasts with the fact that all of these programs have a required course in pediatrics, even though less than 2% of nurses work in pediatrics when they graduate. Almost 60% of all baccalaureate nursing programs have no faculty member specifically prepared in geriatrics (Mezey, 2002).

In nursing, the practice is that if you provide care for older people, you are by definition a Geriatric Nurse, and the same holds true for physicians and social workers. Many of the 2.2 million nurses do take specialized training in specific areas such as oncology, cardiovascular nursing, and perioperative nursing, but although most of the patients that nurses take care of within these fields are older patients, very few of the nurses are trained and experienced in the art and the science of care of older adults. The American Nursing Association estimates that only a little over 12,500 nurses have specialized training in geriatrics (Mezey, 2002).

There is a second level of more specialized nursing, Advanced Practice Nurses or Nurse Practitioners. Nurse Practitioners are Masters prepared nurses who are trained in a particular area and are recognized as Adult Nurse Practitioners, Family Nurse Practitioners, or Geriatric Nurse Practitioners. They are prepared to work alongside their physician and social work colleagues with a specialization in health prevention and illness management. They can prescribe medications, including controlled substances, in almost all states and they work under an individual license that allows them to practice both independently and interdependently. There are about 50,000 practicing Nurse Practitioners who are certified at a national level but of these only about 5,500 are certified in geriatrics as Geriatric Nurse Practitioners.

The number of Nurse Practitioners specializing in geriatrics is very small, but the nursing profession has recently initiated a major effort to assure that nurses who graduate as Adult Nurse Practitioners and Family Nurse Practitioners do acquire a specialization in care of older adults. They are exposed to geriatric content through required courses, and schools are being encouraged to require geriatric clinical experience as well. Many of the educational programs focus not only on nursing care of the frail elderly but on care of well older adults by offering experiences in senior centers and in settings where older adults live independently, such as naturally occurring retirement communities, thus broadening their experiences from the sick elderly to how older people live their lives beyond an average 5.7 days they spend in a hospital per annum. The nursing profession has introduced geriatric content that exposes students to care of the chronically ill elderly in their own homes as well as to older adults and how they function.

Educational nursing programs teach nurses how to view their practice both theoretically at the classroom level and via role models in the clinical setting. The current geriatric nursing perspective that is taught may fit well with what the Baby Boomers wish to experience when they grow old (Mezey, 2002). For instance, nurses are taught the following:

- The nurse's role with the patient should be temporary.
- The nurse's goal is to help the patient gain control over his/her own health. This fits with the Baby Boomers' wish to retain control of their care.
- Nurses take a holistic approach to care.
- Nurses take an interdisciplinary approach to care.
- The nurse's objective is to help the patient to attain, retain, and regain health.
- There is less a focus on diagnosis of health problems but rather an emphasis on management of and living with an illness. This approach is crucial when caring for persons suffering from chronic health conditions and requiring long-term care.

Today's educational directions are in preventing illness, managing the consequences of a disease, and, where appropriate, helping people achieve a peaceful death. These objectives are the hallmarks of good geriatric nursing care. Nurses are particularly effective in their practice when they are engaged in giving immunizations, promoting health, or improving adherence to a treatment plan, whether that be medications, diet, or exercise. This includes patient and family education, advising people about what treatment options to choose, and helping people think about advanced care planning.

Geriatric nurses are particularly well prepared for working in teams, which is essential when caring for older persons because no one professional has all the knowledge and skills to be able to meet their multiple, long-term care needs. In the education of Nurse Practitioners, the goal is to prepare them to be particularly skilled and to contribute to the team in the areas of functional assessment and mental health capacity The management of adherence to medication and treatment regimens and the prevention and treatment of geriatric syndromes (e.g., falls, sleep disturbances, urinary incontinence) are other areas in which to build nursing skills. Given what is being learned of the lifestyles of older persons and the cultural diversity among them, educators are introducing additional areas of education.

SOCIAL WORK EDUCATION

A common theme among gerontological social work educators is "the existence of an aging society (now and in our future) necessitating an increased pool of well-trained gerontological social workers and the inevitable demands this has on professional education" (Mellor & Ivry, 2002, p. 3). The social work profession, like the other professions, is severely lacking in numbers of gerontological/geriatric specialists. There are nearly 600,000 self-identified social workers in the United States, although the American Association of State Social Work Boards notes that only about 320,000 social work licenses have been issued, meaning that over half of all social workers are unlicensed. Only 5,000 of the 155,000 members of the National Association of Social Workers report that aging is their primary area of practice (Rosen & Zlotnik, 2001). No national certification for gerontological social work exists so it is difficult to estimate how many social workers have actually received training for work with older persons. However, it is probably safe to assume that the numbers are inadequate to meet the need and that too few social workers are trained in gerontological social work. This is so, even though a NASW survey of its members, undertaken almost

15 years ago, revealed that 62% of its respondents who were not specializing in aging nevertheless indicated that they required aging knowledge in their practice (Peterson & Wendt, 1990). More recently, the John A. Hartford Foundation, as part of its geriatric social work initiative, funded the CSWE/SAGE-SW Competencies Project.* A literature search and an expert panel resulted in the identification of 65 content items relevant to geriatric social work from the three learning domains of knowledge of older persons and their families, professional skills, and professional practice. A survey of 2,400 practitioners and educators was then undertaken to determine what gerontological/geriatric knowledge and skills are required in practice. Respondents were asked which competencies all social workers need and which relate to specialized practice required only by advanced practitioners in aging. The resulting data indicate "that over one-half of the 65 aging competencies included in the survey were ones thought to be needed by all social workers" (Rosen & Zlotnik, 2001).

The current challenge to the profession lies in recruiting students into practice in the aging field and ensuring that they receive classroom education as well as field work experiences that provide them with the knowledge and skills they need to work with older persons and their families. The Council on Social Work Education notes that only 16% of social work programs offer a gerontology specialization (Rosen & Zlotnik, 2001). Like medicine and nursing, the social work profession is now benefiting from the federal HRSA initiatives and foundation support, most notably from the John A. Hartford Foundation and the Hearst Foundation, programs that develop faculty leadership in aging and offer focused class/practicum experiences for Master level social work students. Aging, as a specialty, is becoming recognized and promoted within the schools of social work and a cohort of faculty is emerging. In addition, the schools of social work are beginning to integrate aging content throughout their core courses with the goal of familiarizing all students with gerontological issues.

At the national level, social work organizations are increasingly focusing on gerontological social work, the work force crisis, and new designs needed for effective service delivery (Briar-Lawson, 2002). Consultants preparing a background paper for the Hartford initiatives advise that, "As the focus of health care changes dramatically toward outpatient

---

*CSWE—Council of Social Work Education and SAGE-SW—the Society for Advancement of Gerontological Education in Social Work.

community-based care for complex health and mental health situations, gerontological social work must expand its focus of concern and articulate a new vision for the profession" (Berkman, Silverstone, & Simmons, 1998, p. 28). Professional organizations and associations have interest groups and committees focused on social work with the aged. Dr. Briar-Lawson notes that social work involves both clinical interventions at the individual level (micro) and work with systems (macro) that foster policy, capacity building, and organizational change. In the past, much of the context of social work has been centered on the family system. Working now to mobilize services and social supports for our aging population, "we recognize that the aging family must be the context for our work. Not only do we have fewer family members to provide elder care, but we may have two or three caregiving crises all within a geriatric intergenerational family system" with the same caregivers caring for parents, grandparents, and possibly for disabled siblings or children. Consequently, social work is developing a new conceptual framework, "from family and from aging, to aging families" (Briar-Lawson, 2002).

Practice-based studies are essential to bring clearer understanding of Baby Boomers' needs, expectations, and hopes, and in the creation of new systems of care. A critical factor in whether the schools of social work will succeed in imparting the needed gerontological knowledge and skills is the development of new field placements. One obstacle in recruiting students into aging as their field of practice has been overcoming their fears that their gerontological social work roles will not be challenging. These new field placements will offer students challenging experiences across the diverse realm of old age, enabling them to work with the well and the frail, representing varying income groups and ethnicities, in exciting and high impact roles (Briar-Lawson, 2002).

Dr. Katherine Briar-Lawson identifies the following areas to be taught within our schools of social work:

- *Knowledge about gerontology:* The new conceptual framework of the aging family includes a shift from solely a disease model to one that focuses on the entire range of need/care, presenting models of healthy aging as well as that of the frail. The majority of Baby Boomers, when reaching old age, will present as active, independent individuals. Society is already redefining the retirement years to factor in this independence. Social workers need to be prepared for a society in which second careers, volunteerism, income planning for old-old age, and great grandparenting exist as counterpoint to those older persons requiring long-term care.

- *New values and ethics:* This educational objective will require faculty to address bias regarding age and disability, gender relevant supports for caregivers, medical decision making, and end-of-life care. These areas all involve value based decisions linked to the social work professional code of ethics.

- *Professional competence in knowledge:* This includes biological/psychological/social aspects of aging; age-relevant policies; barriers to effective outcomes; medical, legal, consumer, and spiritual issues.

- *Communication skills at all levels:* This means one-on-one, group, family, as well as public presentations, testimony, and written articles.

- *Assessment and intervention skills:* These skills need to be learned at the clinical as well as at the policy and systems level.

- *Intergenerational understanding:* Focusing on the aging family, social workers need to assess intergenerational care capacity and recognize intergenerational patterns of behavior. For instance, if child abuse and neglect occurs, "there is a 50% chance that there will be domestic violence and when we see domestic violence there may be a 50% chance of elder abuse or neglect" (Briar-Lawson, 2002). The same may be true for substance abuse, mental health syndromes, and health risk factors. The research and databases on these social problems are unconnected but this must change as we strive to think and practice within an intergenerational framework.

- *Cultural competence:* Our older population is culturally diverse and will become even more so with the aging of the Baby Boomers. Cultural competence is both a knowledge and a skill area that is vital for every social worker engaged with the aging family and must be included within the social work curriculum.

- *Interprofessional skills:* Older persons may have multiple systems and service providers serving them. If we wish to integrate the services and care provided, we must be interprofessional in our practices. Interprofessionalism means increased collaboration in practice and new paradigms for service delivery. Interagency task forces and interest groups that bring members of different delivery service networks together to work on common issues are examples of sound interprofessionalism (e.g., collaboration between the aging network and the mental retardation/developmentally disabled network (MR/DD) which has led to Memorandums of Understanding regarding service delivery at the national, state, and city levels, and the collaboration between the aging and HIV/AIDS networks, which has resulted in a national association with free-standing local groups in many states).

- *Interdisciplinary skills:* Much of social work is interdisciplinary in nature and especially so in work with the older frail population for whom medical, environmental, legal, and social issues are intertwined. The training of social work students needs to include preparation for effective work within the interdisciplinary setting. A national team of social workers involved in the Geriatric Interdisciplinary Team Training (GITT) program, funded by the John A. Hartford Foundation, issued a statement in 1998 concerning the social work contributions to the interdisciplinary team. The group states that "social workers with their training in interpersonal relationships, groupwork and (often) interdisciplinary team skills play a vital role in the development and functioning of the interdisciplinary team unit and in all major phases of its work, including assessment, goal setting and care planning, and monitoring/evaluation" (Lindemann & Mellor, 1998). The primary roles filled by social workers in the team on behalf of the older client and the family are identified as: assessor, care manager, counselor, liaison between patient/family and medical profession, advocate, and community resource expert.

"Social work practice and its educational framework must be intergenerational, inter-professional, interdisciplinary and multicultural" (Briar-Lawson, 2002).

The trends and changes occurring in the delivery of health care are challenging the traditional role of social work in health care. This has prompted a number of social work leaders to review current social work education and advise on new content areas to be included in the curriculum, many of which parallel those identified by Dr. Briar-Lawson. Dr. Edward Pecukonis and his co-authors warn that social work in health care is at a critical juncture, and faces an uncertain future. They recommend that social work education include content on the brain and the central nervous system (its influence on behavior), psychopharmacology, health promotion, and disease prevention, and that in this era of increasing medical technology and genetic engineering, social workers gain the knowledge and skills to become ethics consultants and advocates for their clients (Pecukonis, Cornelius, & Parrish, 2003). The New York Academy of Medicine study, mentioned earlier, drew several implications for social work training from its findings, which, while applicable to all social workers in health care, are particularly relevant to health care social work with older persons. The study found that the health care trends identified above are resulting in a growing team-based approach; an increased need for case management; emphasis on health promotion and disease prevention; attention to critical path models and solution-focused therapy; increased need for patient education related to health care coverage and financing; and attention to patient outcomes, research and evaluation of social work services (Volland et al., 2000).

Also of interest is the finding that population-specific social work practice will be increasingly important (Volland, 2000), due to the climate of rationed resources plus a growing tendency to view the patient holistically as a member of family and community systems, and, potentially, a recipient of services from two or more service delivery systems. In the aging literature these specific populations are identified as special populations of older persons—the developmentally disabled, those with HIV/AIDS, the dually diagnosed of mentally ill and chemically dependent, and so forth (Mellor, 1996).

As a result of these new demands on social workers, the study authors identified three sets of social work skills that need to be stressed in the curriculum of social work schools in order to enhance social work practice and prepare social workers for the future. These are:

> *Basic skills*, including interviewing and assessment techniques that retain biopsychosocial emphasis but incorporate standardized screening measures; data management; setting of goal-based outcomes; and application of analytic skills to evaluate data and outcomes.
>
> *Population-specific skills*, including knowledge of racial, ethnic, and cultural characteristics of a population; knowledge of treatment modalities appropriate to the patient's social situation; and knowledge of terminology, policies, regulations, and ways to access systems of care specific to the disease or population in question.
>
> *Autonomy-building skills*, including the ability to assist in securing grants and other financial resources; enhanced training in making ethical decisions; knowledge of program and finance management; ability to help patients and families negotiate health care systems; and training in interdisciplinary collaboration, conflict mediation,

and advocacy within the health care setting and in the larger arena of health care legislation and regulation (Volland, 2000).

MEDICAL EDUCATION

Although a high percentage of physicians' patients are over 65 years of age, fewer than 9,000 physicians are Board certified in geriatrics. Less than 15 percent of psychiatrists reporting a high geriatric patient ratio had completed the certificate for qualification in geriatric psychiatry by 1999 (Halpain, Harris, McClure, & Jeste, 1999).

The American Geriatrics Society estimates that more than 36,000 geriatricians will be needed in the coming years and yet medical students, like nursing students, are ill prepared in geriatric medicine. Only three of the country's 145 allopathic and osteopathic schools of medicine have a department of geriatrics, and only 14 schools include geriatrics among their required courses, resulting in fewer than 3% of all medical students taking a course in geriatrics. Yet, it is known that older persons tend to use health care services more than younger adults (O'Neill & Barry, 2003). Over two thirds of hospitalized patients are over 65 years of age and, in the community, older persons make almost 25% of all office visits (National Center for Health Statistics). The Health Related Services Administration (HRSA) of the federal government is spearheading continuing education related to geriatric care for the medical profession and other disciplines through funding of Geriatric Education Centers and a number of foundations support fellowships in geriatric training and geriatric educational projects.

Dr. Adelman projected a more future-oriented educational program for medical students that he believes will make them responsive to the health care needs of the Baby Boomers when this generation reaches its older years (Adelman, 2002). Dr. Adelman's educational guidelines are as follows.

- Medical students must first *examine their own attitudes toward aging*. The U.S. is an ageist society in which it is unglamorous to be old and medicine mirrors this societal ageism that makes denial of aging easy with the advent of Botox, Viagra, plastic surgery, and childbirth in one's fifties. The medical student must face his/her own ageism and understand the myths about aging. Destructive false beliefs about older people may undermine a physician's care of older patients.

- Medical students must recognize that *aging is not synonymous with illness*. Successful aging does not necessarily mean being able to bungee jump and skateboard, but is about maintaining function. This is what the medical profession terms "adaptive competence," referring to the individual's capacity to respond with resilience to physical, psychosocial, or environmental changes that occur later in life. Medical students should further understand the benefits of health promotion and disease prevention at any age. Weightlifting and strength-building exercises are as beneficial for 95-year-olds as for younger persons.

- Medical students need to *learn age-specific screening measures* to detect disease at an early stage. And, perhaps even more important, they need to understand tertiary prevention—how chronic diseases, such as emphysema or coronary artery disease, can be managed to improve functioning and prevent future decline.

- Medical students must learn that *cognitive decline, depression, urinary incontinence,* and other elements that we view today as components of aging are actually *not part of normal aging* and must be assessed carefully and then treated with rigorous and aggressive interventions.

- Medical students must become *aware of the ageist beliefs* and tendencies exhibited by the Baby Boomers themselves. Ageism can have a dangerously personal focus unlike other isms (racism, sexism, etc.) where the object of discrimination is another person. If individuals hold ageist beliefs and are fortunate enough to survive to old age, they become the object of their own discrimination. Ageist beliefs by an aging boomer may well sabotage successful aging.

- It is important that medical students *understand the heterogeneous nature of the older population* and experience non-frail, community-residing, robust, and productive elderly. Most medical students are exposed to hospitalized elderly who are the frailest subset and this contributes to a biased perspective of aging. The students need older people as faculty and role models, and they need to be exposed to intergenerational relationships and activities.

- Medical students need to *be prepared to be health educators*. It is estimated that about 44% of today's older population lack the most basic reading skills necessary for full functioning, such as taking medicines, keeping appointments, preparing for medical tests, and giving adequate informed consent. Advancing the cause of health literacy is pivotal in ensuring that our future older patients are successful partners in the management of their own care.

• It is also critical for all medical students to be fully *cognizant of the fundamentals of geriatric medicine,* that is, to be superb internists. Geriatrics encompasses all the diseases that an internist sees but it can be complicated as an older individual often presents with multiple diseases and, as a result, multiple interacting medications. It is important that students understand drug use and interactions with the elderly as well as the geriatric syndromes—falls, osteoporosis, delirium, depression, and so forth—that can be exacerbated by medications.

• Medical students must *recognize that medical and psychosocial factors can conspire to impair function* and, recognizing this, utilize an interdisciplinary approach. An example is an 88-year-old woman, who was about to be evicted from her home. Her blood pressure was wildly high and she needed to be started on medicines which, as a side effect, affected her balance. Her home situation was chaotic. The social worker at the clinic was able to deal with the eviction notice and secure home care. The patient's blood pressure went down. The physician was then able to take the patient off her medicines and normal homeostasis was regained.

• Medical students must *learn about the reality of living with a chronic illness.* Today, over 100 million Americans experience chronic medical or mental illness and by 2020 this will increase to 134 million individuals. Medical students need to comprehend what it is like to be confronted with a chronic illness with the accompanying fears of loss of independence, of identity, of physical comfort, and even of life itself. At the same time, students need to understand that a 90-year-old with hypertension, spinal stenosis, hearing problems, coronary artery disease, high cholesterol, Paget's disease and a newly placed pacemaker can still lead an independent and fulfilling life. Students need to understand that chronic illness does not mean the end of life. On the contrary, the focus is on the ability to function. Assisting a patient to cope with chronic illness may not be as glamorous as life-saving surgery but students can learn that it provides incredible rewards and satisfaction and is just as significant and crucial to the patient and the family.

- *Communication* is a vital content area in medical curriculum. Medicine has a history of paternalism with patients, which does not bode well for medicine's relationship with the Baby Boomers and their expectations of an emphasis on patient empowerment, shared ownership of information, and self-management of care. There needs to be a patient-centered model of interaction, or partnership, between physician and patient. Students need to learn to empower their patients and to understand the significance and the power of communication in geriatric medicine. Research shows that the quality of the patient/physician relationship deeply influences a patient's adherence to medication and other treatments, affecting the patient's health status and satisfaction. Competency in a wide range of areas depends on the acquisition of strong communication skills. For example, patients are generally overwhelmed and threatened by questions in assessment of memory and cognition, but by using sensitive communication skills, the physician can make the experience less threatening. Often the older patient is accompanied by relatives and there may be several people involved in the medical encounter. It is apparent from reviews of such physician/patient interaction that the physician tends to talk to an accompanying relative, often a daughter, leaving the patient out of the scenario. The students need to know about communication both in small groups and one-on-one. Physicians need to allow patients to be able to present themselves within the medical encounter. Situations of elder abuse and certain other confidential issues may never be identified unless there is time spent alone with that older person. And, finally, strong communication skills are required in times of death and dying, to be able to assess the wishes of the patient and family, to help them communicate with each other, and to become comfortable in facing death.

- Communication skills are also required in *working with other members of the health care team*. Medical students and medical residents need to learn how to use social, environmental, and psychosocial information in diagnosis and treatment and how to work collaboratively with other health disciplines. Being a team member does not come naturally and this has never been part of a student's training.

- Medical students need to *understand the importance of the culture and values* of their patients and to be receptive to the family structures they will encounter. Understanding the culture and values of an individual is pivotal in any kind of relationship and the physician/patient relationship is no exception (Diaz, 2002).

- Medical students today also *require technological communication skills.* Baby Boomers are a computer literate generation, providing an opportunity for increased communication and growth of the doctor/patient relationship. Students must learn how to use e-mail appropriately, to be able to e-mail information in a form that the patient can read and understand, and to identify and advise on websites that give reliable information to older people, recognizing that patients may have turned to the Internet and technology for information even before seeking professional advice. There are other communication opportunities in the world of electronics, such as telemedicine for use with the homebound. Medical students must be technically adept and skillful in making diagnoses and developing treatment plans through use of the new technology.

- Medical students need to become *knowledgeable about alternative/complementary medicine.* Fifteen percent of the hospitals in the U.S. are creating complementary medicine sites that conduct yoga, stress reduction, massage, exercise, and nutrition classes. Forty-three percent of Americans utilize alternative medicine, so it behooves medical students to learn the appropriate use of these complementary therapies (e.g., that acupuncture can ease nausea and pain, tai chi can help in balance disorders, biofeedback can be helpful with urinary incontinence). Students need to be informed and able to analyze the literature, to use critical thinking when reviewing data to determine whether an alternative therapy is justified or not.

- Medical students need to *understand the role of psychiatry* and to gain skills in recognizing psychosocial issues. The practice of medicine with older persons requires the ability to recognize mental health problems in both older patients and/or family members and other caregivers. Furthermore, the prevalence of psychiatric illness (depression, dementia) among older people necessitates a robust curriculum in mental health for present and future students.

- Medical students need *knowledge of community service agencies and types of specialists* that they can refer to when they encounter problems beyond their knowledge base. Once they have graduated and are practicing, this learning can be related to identifying specific services and specialists within their geographic environment.

- *Environmental geriatrics* is an emerging field to which medical students need to be exposed. Environmental geriatrics examines the interaction between the environment and the health condition of the patient. It includes looking at age-appropriate design of the patient's surroundings and seeking environmentally responsive changes toward the goal of maintaining or regaining independence (e.g., enabling older people to bathe independently, or improving mobility with ergonomic, metrically designed handrails, etc.).

- It is critical for medical students to *engage in research* that relates to the basic biology of aging and applied gerontological issues and ask questions such as, Does telephone reassurance actually decrease the sense of isolation or decrease the amount of depression experienced by an older patient? As a profession, physicians need to document interventions that work (Adelman, 2002, used with permission).

Dr. Adelman believes that the end result of including all the above in medical school curricula would be the development of the kind of doctors that he, as a Baby Boomer himself, wants in his future. The kind of doctor Dr. Adelman envisages is:

Someone who knows me well, has a sense of my identity and even likes me, and cares about me, and whom I can trust. Someone who is adept in medicine; keeps up-to-date; is completely conversant with aging issues and geriatric medicine; and someone who is flexible, creative, and can think out of the box. Someone who has a belief in my future, and understands my potential to age well, and will assist me in this goal, and wants to work with me as a partner. Someone who knows how to share information—both interpersonally/face-to-face, as well as electronically. Someone who knows his or her limits, knows when to refer to other disciplines, knows when I should see a social worker, knows when I should see a nurse, and believes in me as a person, not merely as a patient, and understands community resources. If necessary, this doctor will refer me to other geri-friendly physicians, subspecialists who are also knowledgeable in aging-related concerns. Someone who can follow me through the continuum of care, someone who will visit me if I'm hospitalized and if I'm in a nursing home for rehabilitation, check in with me there as well. Someone who can advocate for me if I become frail, a physician who has the skills to maintain my function and someone whom I can trust if I need a paternalistic intervention, if my capacity for appropriate decision-making is compromised or divorced from reality. Someone who will understand my wishes and will abide by them and someone who will be there to help me die well, who will have interpersonal depth and some spiritual acumen and who can assist my loved ones as I die and when I die. [Adelman, 2002]

SUMMARY

Any analysis of health care for older persons today focuses on two major issues: the scarcity of appropriately educated health care professionals and the multiple changes experienced in delivery of health care.

First, there are insufficient numbers of health care professionals with the knowledge and skills to meet the care needs of the current older population. This shortage will become even more pronounced as the numbers of older persons begin to escalate by the end of the decade. Unless we can rapidly overcome this disparity in demand and supply, there will be a serious lack of health care professionals with the knowledge and skills to provide appropriate health care to the Baby Boomers when they grow old.

It is apparent in looking back over the last thirty years that many discoveries in health care knowledge and changes in its delivery have occurred and continue to surface. These changes have resulted in a new knowledge base for health care professionals that has reshaped their perceptions of the elderly. New discoveries and new modalities of care continue to emerge. Planning for tomorrow requires tomorrow's aging population, the Baby Boomers, to join the health care professionals today in presenting their expectations and fashioning a future to meet them.

Baby Boomers as health care consumers can be a major force in shaping the delivery of health care in the future. Baby Boomers can keep health care professionals focused on needs and expectations so that, as a society, we continue to move toward a patient-centered, holistic approach delivered by interdisciplinary teams in the community. Simultaneously, it is hoped that the current advances in training and educating health care professionals to engage in this new mode of care will gain momentum and, potentially, attract more students into the field.

The Baby Boomers are recognized as informed and proactive consumers of health care; however, they express doubt that a comprehensive patient-centered care model will be available to them in their older years. This proactive stance can enable Baby Boomers, as they approach old age, to utilize and maximize health care benefits for their older relatives and secure the kind of health care system that they desire for their own future. Without the pressure and advocacy from Baby Boomers, health care consumers, practitioners, and educators could easily slip back into their normal modes of practice.

The projections of the health care professionals as reported here could be the beginning of deliberations between health care providers and Baby Boomers. It is the task of the health care professionals to listen to the Baby Boomers and plan accordingly and the task of the Baby Boom generation to be vocal and explicit in continually reminding practitioners and educators on how health care is to be delivered (Mezey, 2002).

REFERENCES

AARP. (2002, May). *Beyond 50:02: A report to the nation on trends in health security.* Washington, DC: Author.

AARP/International Longevity Center. (2003). *Unjust desserts: Financial realities of older women.* Washington, DC: Author.

Adelman, R. (2002, April 24). Looking ahead: Educating Geriatricians for the future. Presentation at Second Summit Meeting: *Can my eighties be like my fifties?* The New York Academy of Medicine, New York.

Berkman, B., Silverstone, B., & Simmons, W. J. (1998). *Social work gerontological practice: The need and strategic proposals for professional development.* Paper prepared for the John A. Hartford Foundation. New York, NY.

Briar-Lawson, K. (2002, April 24). Looking ahead: Educating social workers for the future. Presentation at Second Summit Meeting: *Can my eighties be like my fifties?* The New York Academy of Medicine, New York.

Diaz, M. (2002, April 24). Looking ahead: Health care for Baby Boomers. Presentation at Second Summit Meeting: *Can my eighties be like my fifties?* The New York Academy of Medicine, New York.

Halpain, M., Harris, J., McClure, F. & Jeste, D. (1999). Training in geriatric mental health: Needs and strategies. *Psychiatric Services, 50*(9), 1205–1208.

Jacoby, S. (2003, May). The nursing squeeze. *AARP Bulletin,* p. 6.

Lindemann, D., & Mellor, M. J. (1998). The role of the social worker in interdisciplinary geriatric teams. *Journal of Gerontological Social Work, 30*(3/4), 3–7.

Mellor, M. J. (1996). Special populations among older persons. In M. J. Mellor (Ed.), *Special aging populations and systems linkages* (pp. 1–10). Binghamton, NY: Haworth.

Mellor, M. J., & Ivry, J. (2002). Introduction to section I. In M. J. Mellor & J. Ivry (Eds.), *Advancing gerontological social work education* (pp. 3–5). New York: Haworth.

Mezey, M. (2002, April 24). Looking ahead: Educating nurses for the future. Presentation at Second Summit Meeting: Can my eighties be like my fifties? The New York Academy of Medicine, New York.

O'Neill, G., & Barry, P. (2003). Training physicians in geriatric care: Responding to critical need. *Public Policy and Aging Report, 13*(2), 17–21. National Academy on an Aging Society. The Gerontological Society of America.

Pecukonis, E., Cornelius, L., & Parrish, M. (2003). The future of health social work. *Social Work in Health Care, 37*(3), 1–15.

Peterson, D. A., & Wendt, P. F. (1990). Employment in the field of aging: A survey of professionals in four fields. *The Gerontologist, 30*, 679–684.

Rosen, A. L., & Zlotnik, J. L. (2001). Social work's response to the growing older population. *Generations. Who Will Care for Older People? Workforce Issues in a Changing Society, 25*(1), 69–71.

Solomon, D., Steel, K., Williams, T. F., Brown, A. S., Brummel-Smith, K., Buirgess, L., et al. (1988). National Institute of Health consensus development conference statement: Geriatric assessment methods for clinical decision making. *Journal of American Geriatric Society, 36*, 342–347.

Volland, P., Berkman, B., Stein, G., & Vaghy, A. (2000). *Social work education for practice in health care. Final report.* New York: The New York Academy of Medicine.

Chapter 12

Community Collaboration and Advocacy

> We know what we want, but we don't know how to get it.
>
> Discussion Group Member
> at Summit # 1

The majority of Baby Boomers appear to give some thought to their retirement years in reference to financial security and the income they will need. Those who can afford to do so are paying into employment-related pension plans or 401(k)s. However, there is a noted lack of retirement planning on their part in reference to potential health care needs, coverage, and costs. Baby Boomers, for the most part, will live longer in good health than preceding generations, but age-related diseases will still remain the lot of many and Baby Boomers should still expect to experience some years of living with chronic disease.

Economists and health care professionals working with older persons are acutely aware of the potential for disaster in the years ahead for the delivery of available, accessible, affordable, high quality health care services to the large older population. All the forum presenters spoke of the necessity of changing our current health care system to meet these needs and the theme was repeated in the workshop discussions. When alerted to these concerns, Baby Boomers are adamant that they do not want to receive the same kind of health care that their parents and grandparents are receiving. They are clear about what they want from a remodeled health care system, considerations that are mostly lacking in our current system—quality care that is patient and family oriented, accessible, affordable, comprehensive, and community based. But, as one summit meeting participant observed, "We know what we want but we don't know how to get it." In response, many of the presenters spoke of the need for the Baby Boom generation to become involved in advocacy efforts and work with the health care system in collaborative community partnerships. "Through uniting, collaborating, a community can build, enhance, expand existing strengths, assets and resources" (Peterson, 2003). Hence this chapter is devoted to community collaboration—what it is and how to accomplish it.

CURRENT TRENDS IN HEALTH CARE DELIVERY

The health care system has been experiencing substantial changes over the past few years in reaction to newly emerging means of financing care and in response to the struggle of health organizations to remain viable within this changing environment. It is, therefore, an opportune time for the Baby Boom generation to become involved and help mold the system to its requirements for the future. The principle of managed care, with insurance companies and health care maintenance organizations (HMOs) becoming the administrative gatekeepers of health care provision, has removed authority from the practicing health care professionals themselves. At the same time, there has been a shift from acute care to ambulatory care with an increase in one-day walk-in surgery and technical innovations, making care in the home more practical. Hospitals are now reserved for the sickest patients requiring specialized care (Rehr, Rosenberg, & Blumenfield, 1998b).

Care of the acutely ill is high maintenance and costly, factors that are motivating hospitals to reconfigure themselves into multipurpose centers. They are undertaking new programs that aim to be comprehensive and multidisciplinary and that integrate medical and social services within a variety of settings. Today's health setting is "a complex entity with an array of facilities and services, including the medical center, nursing homes, public social service, community, family and child support programs, linkages to employer/employee health arrangements, community based primary care clinics and managed care enterprises, and prevention, fitness, and wellness programs" (Rehr et al., 1998b, p.

168). This description matches much of what the Baby Boomers envisage but there are often essential factors missing, such as true integration of the various services, a continuum of care with an interdisciplinary team of health care professionals staying with each individual patient moving between the levels of care, and a patient/family role in decision making.

Meanwhile, primary care physicians in the community are subjected to management interference in the administration of their practices and are frequently overwhelmed by the regulations and paperwork demanded by insurance companies and the government Medicare program. Primary care physicians are most often unschooled in care of the older patient even though the majority of their patients are likely to be over 65 years of age. A small study undertaken in Nebraska found that primary care physicians surveyed find caring for older patients difficult. This is due not only to the medical complexity and chronic nature of health issues presented by older adults but to the personal and interpersonal challenges that are encountered in the doctor/patient relationship (such as hearing loss, family participation) and the administrative burden of the Medicare regulations (Adams et al., 2002). Much depends on the proportion of older persons within a medical practice. Too many older patients results in too much time and trouble given the financial reimbursement rates. This suggests that primary care physicians are likely to limit the number of older patients for whom they care and, indeed, there is a growing trend across the country of physicians dropping Medicare patients and refusing to take on newly eligible individuals.

Consumers/patients' participation in their own health care, a major element in Baby Boomers' wishes for the future, is already becoming apparent. They are beginning to take responsibility for their health through involvement in preventive activities—exercise, nutrition, stress relief—and, to an even greater extent, are informing themselves about health conditions and treatments via the Internet. But in spite of the written emphasis and advice columns on prevention measures to ensure a healthy old age, health care itself is not yet fully geared up for prevention or for health education. Preventive interventions and practices are rarely reimbursable (Rehr et al., 1998b). Health education from someone with medical knowledge and personal knowledge of the individual patient is sparse even though of vital importance, especially as most of the information available on the world wide web is generic, frequently biased in a given direction, or easily misinterpreted.

Long-term care of persons managing chronic health conditions is the essence of health care for the older person. It is this area, above all else, that requires innovative and creative changes to ensure it meets the hoped-for standards set by the Baby Boomers. Kane (2003) states that problems with our existing long-term care for seniors are twofold. "First help is irregularly available and difficult to arrange and sustain in the settings that seniors prefer, at the time and in the manner they wish, in the amounts they need, and at the price they (or subsidizing governments) can afford. Second and conversely, care in the places of greatest access and public subsidy, that is, in nursing homes, too often comes at the hideous prices of loss of dignity, freedom, privacy, and a meaningful life." These problems are exactly those the Baby Boomers wish to be rid of and should set about changing with all the advocacy efforts they can muster.

Current issues of access to health care, rationing, and the ethics of promoting costly procedures for older persons at the expense of younger patients are likely to become even more crucial as the Baby Boomers reach their older years. Because the older population will constitute such a high percentage of all patients and because this population will overwhelmingly present with chronic illness needs and functional disabilities, there will be a basic shift from diagnostic care that characterizes the acute care patient to that of functional assessment with a focus on social risk factors. Third party insurance, whether private or government based, will be sought to cover medical, nursing, and social aspects of integrated and selectively allocated care (Rehr et al., 1998b).

COMMUNITY COLLABORATION

A continuum of health care delivery has been an acknowledged objective for the last fifty years. Furthermore, it has long been recognized that the achievement of such an objective requires strong community–agency relationships and, with this in mind, liaisons between health care institutions (hospitals, clinics, etc.) and community agencies have been forged since the 1980s (Rehr, Blumenfield, & Rosenberg, 1998a). Social workers in the health care arena are particularly interested in collaboration as a tool to effect the integration of social and medical care under the rubric of health care. As Bess Dana noted over twenty years ago, collaboration is "one means through which social work makes its values, knowledge and skills felt in the formulation of social health policy, the governance of social health services, and the study and treatment of health and medical care problems in individuals and population groups" (Dana, 1983).

Dana's statement applies equally to nursing and medicine. Since it was written there has been increasing interest in interdisciplinary teamwork within health care of older persons. The National Institutes of Health held a Consensus Development Conference in 1987 and put forth a strong statement in favor of interdisciplinary teamwork/ collaboration as the most effective means of assessing and treating older persons with health problems (Solomon et al., 1988). Since then, there has been a continuing stream of literature on the development of interdisciplinary teams. Lessons learned from building health care teams across disciplines—communication, consensus building, re-spect—are applicable to the creation of community-wide collabora-tive activities.

The notion of health and social care for older persons offered through a community-based collaborative arrangement dates back to the early 1980s. At that time, the Centers for Medicare and Medicaid Services supported three demonstration projects, affectionately called SHMOs—Social Health Maintenance Organizations. The goal of the SHMOs was to provide geriatric services and to support primary care through improved coordination among ambulatory care, post-hospital continuity of care, home health, and chronic care providers. The stan-dard Medicare coverage of hospital and physician services was expanded to include additional benefits targeted at those persons at risk for nurs-ing home care. These expanded services included personal and home-maker care, adult day care, respite for caregivers, and even prescription coverage, home modifications, and emergency response systems. Also included were risk identification and prevention programs (Newcomer, Harrington, & Kane, 2002). Older persons, under Medicare waivers, contracted with the SHMOs and received health and social services that enabled them to manage chronic health conditions and remain in the community. Development of the SHMOs required community collabo-ration. These demonstration projects have now been transitioned into Medicare+Choice plans.

The second generation of this social health care demonstration was launched in 1996 with the Health Plan of Nevada as its prototype. Coordination is undertaken at all levels of care and ambulatory care management teams (ACMs) are established that are responsible for patient care planning, starting at an individual's enrollment in the plan with health screening and assessments and continuing with care planning and the coordination and access to community services as indicated. Coordination is further strengthened by interdisciplinary team meetings between members of the Geriatrics Department and the ACMs. Although this model takes a long time to implement, it results in increased physician use and lower emergency room use (Newcomer et al., 2002).

Such plans are by no means universal. Even though many medical centers have moved toward community collaborative efforts with the objective to provide social health services at the community level with health education and screening, there is limited commitment by managed care to public health. This means that medical centers often lack the resources to continue their community collaborative objectives (Rehr et al., 1998b). Proponents of community collaboration believe that simultaneously the capacity of communities to help themselves has declined. This, they suggest, is due to the complexity of issues that any one community faces, the need for specialized knowledge to deal with these complex issues, and an inability of redistributive policies to deal with inequality (Peterson, 2003).

In spite of the difficulties, health institutions and organizations must relate to their communities to remain viable by any standards. Access or lack of access may "easily be the most important dynamic, affecting users and providers" (Peake, Brenner, & Rosenberg, 1998). In addition to the current barrier of complexity, barriers to community collaboration are control and territorialism (protecting turf) and lack of communication. These same barriers are identified as issues in the development of interdisciplinary health care teams. The health of older adults, as with children and disabled adults, results from the interplay of psychological, social, biological, and environmental factors (Dana, 1983). Because of this, the interdisciplinary health care team with members of various disciplines including, ideally, the patient and family, is the most appropriate modality for assessment and care. Each member/discipline contributes from his/her specialized perspective. Though each of the parts is critical, they are contributed in the context of the whole; thus the whole becomes greater than its parts. This is also true of collaboration at the wider level of the community. This sharing of perspectives and agendas from a range of community activists and organizations leads to effective solutions to problems.

For the most part, and despite the overall sweeping changes wrought by managed care and third party reimbursement strategies, health care of the older individual patient follows the traditional medical model. Suggested changes include participation of "nurse case managers in primary care practice; programs that facilitate communication between families and staff in primary care, similar to such programs in the nursing home setting; simplification of Medicare documentation and increased reimbursement; improvement of community resources to meet needs of the chronically ill; changes in medical education" to include more geriatric training (Adams et al., 2002). Some of these changes can be initiated within the primary care practice and hospital settings but others require involvement with the community. Rehr and colleagues (1998b) suggest a system of community service centers available to all community residents that are comprehensive, accessible, and accountable. Medical centers today have many of the necessary resources but they need to be enhanced and a system established that becomes a vital link between the medical centers and their communities as well as between the various services/units within the medical centers themselves.

MODELS OF COMMUNITY COLLABORATION

What form any one community collaborative effort takes will depend on the identified needs and the community itself. There are a variety of models in existence. One of the earliest examples of health care organization and community collaboration for purposes of providing comprehensive care, even prior to the SHMOs, was the On Lok SeniorHealth agency in San Francisco, founded in 1971. On Lok's mission is to help frail elderly people live an independent life outside the nursing home. It pioneered the integration of medical and social care for older persons in the community and relies heavily on interdisciplinary teams to determine and carry out the care plans. OnLok SeniorHealth became the model for Programs of All-inclusive Care for the Elderly (PACE), which model was tested via demonstration projects in the 1980s and became permanent when authorized by the Balanced Budget Act of 1997. The PACE programs provide and coordinate all needed preventive, primary, acute, and long-term care services so that older persons can continue living in the community. A multidisciplinary team approach in an adult day care center is used and supplemented by in-home and referral services. Today, there are 40 PACE programs in existence throughout the U.S.

Other models of collaboration exist between health organizations and colleges and housing programs for seniors such as congregate housing, assisted living, and naturally occurring retirement centers (NORCs). These programs allow care to be delivered in the community setting while also serving the dual purpose of providing teaching opportunities and role models for students. Yet other models involve auxiliary boards of community members attached to hospitals and medical centers as community sounding boards and advisory groups. Finally, with the proliferation of self-help groups during the '80s and '90s, health care organizations are frequently involved in reaching out to the community on behalf of self-help groups that they either sponsor directly or use as referral resources for their patients.

WHY COLLABORATE?

The driving force behind a health organization's interest in building collaborative relationships with its surrounding community may be the desire to integrate services, to reduce duplicative costs and/or to build a reputation that attracts customers. In reality it is probably a mix of all three objectives. The vision of health care held by the Baby Boomers requires health care organizations to collaborate with community resources and to plan collegially alongside patients and families. But before this stage is reached, Baby Boomers, advocating for the kind of health care they want available to them, should seek to collaborate at the local and national levels with representatives of the existing health care system (i.e., hospital and HMO administrators, home care and nursing facility staff, primary care physicians, Medicare and private insurance agents). Becoming involved now will enable them to help shape the health care system of the future for their own future.

The relationship between the consumer and providers in interaction is the most critical factor in achieving mutually desired outcomes (Rehr et al., 1998b). This is true for all areas of commerce but is of particular significance for the development and delivery of health care which is of crucial importance to the individual patient and family. Yet providers rarely interact with consumers in the planning stages, let alone at the point of delivery. The consumer, as an ambulatory or hospitalized patient, is currently viewed, not as a partner with a voice in his/her care, but as a set of symptoms or a disease. This is especially true of the older person. Even the advent of the consumer choice movement and the legislative efforts at the national level for a Patient's Bill of Rights have failed to elevate the patient to the level of the health care providers for purposes of joint decision making. Baby Boomers want to change this.

As long ago as 1970, Dana noted that there are limitations in a hospital-based model addressing the comprehensive care needs of people in their homes and communities. Such care requires appropriate strategies dependent on "active engagement of those with the problem in its assessment and resolution" (Dana, 1983). Collaboration, initiated by Baby Boomers as health care consumers, is thus a necessary and vital intervention.

STEPS IN BUILDING COMMUNITY COLLABORATION

Collaboration at any level is complex. Suzi Kay, referring to building coalitions, reminds us that "coalitions often start with one agency that identifies a problem or a need that is larger than any one organization can address and then uses that topic to convene the group, keeping in mind that the topic or issue will be redefined in the organizing process" (Kay, 2001). Collaboration requires understanding of each other's role, reaching agreement on the problem to be addressed, an ability to engage in the group process, and a sense of self-worth both as an individual practitioner/consumer and as an institution, for those organizations represented at the table (Dana, 1983).

The initial step is to determine which community is to serve as the community of collaboration (see Table 12.1). "A community can be any group of individuals or families working toward a common goal. A community may include but is not limited to: a town, a city, a neighborhood, an office, an industry, a profession, a school, a religion, a corporation, a geographic, or political entity" (Peterson, 2003). Organizations communicate with their community in different ways. They may offer education, seek input/feedback, or engage in damage control. True collaboration goes beyond these forms and implies an equality of authority between the collaborating groups and individuals.

To reach the initial stage of gathering your community around your issue, it is usually necessary for two or three people with a "passion for the purpose" to convene to brainstorm. Occasionally this occurs spontaneously but generally requires the action of one person to call a meeting of two or three like-minded individuals to vocalize the issue/concern and to plan a larger group meeting of invited persons and

TABLE 12.1   The Sense of Community—What Is a Community?

Indicator	Strong Sense of Community	Weak Sense of Community
Sense of membership	The active participants proudly display symbols of membership in the community.	The active participants do not view themselves as a community.
Mutual importance	The active participants recognize, cherish, and support the contributions of each other.	Participants are active only because one or a few powerful persons are involved.
Shared world views	The active participants hold common beliefs and promote shared values important to them.	The active participants hold fundamentally different beliefs and values and cannot reconcile their differences.
Bonding/ networking	The active participants enjoy one another and look forward to time spent together.	The active participants have no affinity for each other and relationships are formal or superficial.
Mutual responsibility for the community	The survival and health of the community is a primary concern of all its active participants.	One or only a few persons struggle to keep the group together.

Source: U.S. Department of Health and Human Services, Center for Substance Abuse Prevention

organizations. It is at this and subsequent meetings that a common cause is defined and members of the collaboration mobilized to take action (see Table 12.2). Capacity to mobilize will vary depending on a number of factors. Table 12.2 identifies those factors that lead to a high level of mobilization on behalf of an issue as well as those that result in a low level of activity and ineffectualness.

Once members and institutions within the community have come together; the common cause or issue has been detailed; and a collaborative entity, with all the hallmarks of high mobilization capacity, has been developed; action to create the desired change(s) can commence. Capacity for action of any single community collaboration effort will also vary, falling along a continuum from strong to weak (see Table 12.3).

A collaborative coalition is likely to be effective when its convenors adopt the following guidelines: obtain a firm commitment from members, remain focused on the mission and plan, communicate with the membership, conduct meaningful meetings, sustain the energy, and

TABLE 12.2 Mobilization Capacity

Indicator	High Mobilization Capacity	Low Mobilization Capacity
Sustained leadership	Strong leaders have emerged to keep activities on track and motivate other community members to stay involved.	The effort is muddling along without leaders who have the qualities to provide direction and motivation.
Formalization	Clear procedures, manuals, ground rules, and role definitions exist to provide a framework for community member participation.	Community members function in an ad hoc manner and newcomers have to define their own roles.
Rewards and incentives	Those involved feel valued and appreciated and receive rewards that make them feel their efforts are worthwhile.	Participants don't feel that they receive rewards that compensate for the cost of their involvement.
Internal and external communication	Active members share experiences and information on a regular basis, and the effort is well covered by local media.	Members rarely communicate with one another outside meetings or contact the media to get coverage of their activities.
Community organizational know-how	A community member with years of successful community organizational experience is actively involved in recruitment and resource mobilization.	The active members are inexperienced at working on a community-based project.
Behind-the-scenes support	A highly effective support team functions to handle day-to-day logistics and provide technical assistance as needed.	Tasks sometimes fall between the cracks or logistics are poorly handled because there is no one specifically responsible for their functions.

Source: U.S. Department of Health and Human Services, Center for Substance Abuse Prevention

maintain good leadership (Kay, 2001). Of course, collaborative efforts can be expected to fluctuate and vary over time and under varying circumstances. A community with a low capacity for action can change to become strong in this area and vice versa. Leaders of a successful community collaboration need to be aware of fluctuations and take the appropriate steps to strengthen capacity for action or, if the original

TABLE 12.3 Readiness for Focused Action

Indicator	High Capacity for Action	Low Capacity for Action
Clarity of goals	The issues facing the community are clear, and consensus exists on the types of responses needed.	There is concern but no consensus regarding the direction for responding.
Feasibility of plan	A practical and flexible action plan is being implemented and updated based on accurate feedback.	The group is muddling through with quick fixes and unrealizable schemes.
Capabilities and resources	The members collectively possess or have access to all needed talents, skills, and resources.	The members have no access to—or are not aware of—the talents, skills, and resources that are needed to mobilize.
Citizen participation and control	The initiative is made up of, and controlled by, members of the targeted community and includes active participation of those most affected by the proposed changes.	There is minimal representation by persons who will be affected by the initiative.
Passion for immediate action	The members are committed to making some positive, goal-directed, and well-conceived change happen in the community as quickly as possible.	The members like to talk, argue, and push their views but are not committed to making some positive change in the community.
High-performance team functioning	The members can function as a high-performance team to get the job done.	The members have a hard time coordinating action and working together.

Source: U.S. Department of Health and Human Services, Center for Substance Abuse Prevention

issue has been resolved, to metamorphose into a new collaborative effort or to disband if the work has been completed. "In a true collaboration, the expectations, degree of collaboration, and sometimes, level of authority, will be negotiated or derived from the collaboration" (Peterson, 2003). If this becomes the case, the value of the community collaboration itself may be sufficient justification for it to be continued, even after the initial objectives have been met. "When creativity, skills, self-efficacy, and motivation accompany collaboration, possibilities are extended, doors are opened, capacity expanded, and success realized" (Peterson, 2003).

Working together to shape a community-based, patient-centered health care system for older persons will benefit all ages, and could become a lasting legacy from the Baby Boom generation to society.

REFERENCES

Adams, W. L., McIlvain, H. E., Lacy, N. L., Magsi, M., Crabtree, B. F., Yenny, S. K., et al. (2002). Primary care for elderly people: Why do doctors find it so hard? *Gerontologist, 42*(6), 835–842.

Dana, B. (1983). The collaborative process. In R. Miller & H. Rehr (Eds.), *Social work issues in health care* (pp. 181–220). Englewood Cliffs, NJ: Prentice Hall.

Kane, R. A. (2003). Book review: Community supports, home care, and long-term services: Looking sideways and backwards for insights on long-term care for older people. *Gerontologist, 43*(2), 274–279.

Kay, S. (2001). Building coalitions. *Center for Medicare Education, Issue Brief, 2*(3), 1–7.

Newcomer, R., Harrington, C., & Kane, R. (2002). Challenges and accomplishments of the second-generation social health maintenance organization. *Gerontologist, 42*(6), 843–852.

Peake, K., Brenner, B., & Rosenberg, G. (1998). Community development and lay participation. In H. Rehr, G. Rosenberg, & S. Blumenfield (Eds.), *Creative social work in health care: Clients, the community, and your organization* (pp. 103–115). New York: Springer.

Peterson, C. R. (2003). Retrieved September 23, 2003, from http://www.community collaboration.net/id20.htm

Rehr, H., Blumenfield, S., Rosenberg, G. (1998a). Collaboration and consultation: Key social work roles in health care. In H. Rehr, G. Rosenberg, & S. Blumenfield (Eds.), *Creative social work in health care: Clients, the community, and your organization* (pp. 93–102). New York: Springer.

Rehr, H., Rosenberg, G., & Blumenfield, S. (1998b). A prescription for social-health care: Responding to the client, the community, and the organization. In H. Rehr, G. Rosenberg, & S. Blumenfield (Eds.), *Creative social work in health care: Clients, the community, and your organization* (pp. 153–181). New York: Springer.

Solomon, D., Steel, K., Williams, T. F., Brown, A. S., Brummel-Smith, K., Buirgess, L., et al. (1988). National Institute of Health consensus development conference statement: Geriatric assessment methods for clinical decision making. *Journal of American Geriatric Society, 36*, 342–347.

U.S. Department of Health and Human Services. (2003). *Effective community mobilization, Lessons from experience*. DHHS, Substance Abuse and Mental Health Services, Administration Center for Substance Abuse Prevention. Retrieved September 30, 2003, from www.communitycollaboration.net/id20.htm

Chapter 13

Can *My Eighties Be Like My Fifties?: Conclusions and Recommendations*

Yes it can, if we as Baby Boomers and health and social service professionals make it happen. And we can.

Summit Participant

INTRODUCTION

The question posed by the Summit series was whether the Baby Boom generation will experience its ninth decade in the same way it experiences its sixth decade. For those in good health with an income that enables them to enjoy safe housing and pursue social, recreational, or educational interests, the question is this: Will their health, income, and lifestyle be similar to that of today and, perhaps most important, will their quality of life remain the same? Certainly those attending the Summit meetings expressed the hope that it would be, although this hope was tempered by recognition of the reality faced by many of today's eighty-year-olds, their parents. For those Baby Boomers already experiencing insufficient income and/or poor health in their fifties, the question to be asked is whether they can expect income, health, and quality of life to improve as they age. Whereas it is anticipated that the majority of future older Americans will remain in good health and

158

financially secure, there will be a considerable number of frail elderly living with physical or mental disabilities, and frequently without the financial resources to obtain the help and care they will need.

During the period of the Summit meetings and the preparation of this publication, a survey, commissioned by AARP, was undertaken to determine what Baby Boomers have to say about their lives and expectations for the future. The findings of this survey indicate that whereas Baby Boomers are "generally upbeat about their future" and "satisfied with their lives overall," they are less satisfied with their personal finances, physical health, leisure activities, and work or career. Baby Boomers want to experience improvements in these areas but just over half of those surveyed think that they are "very likely" to improve their personal finances or physical health. On a more encouraging note, however, the survey also found that Baby Boomers believe that "if they really want to do something, they will find a way to achieve it" (Keegan, Gross, Fisher, & Remez, 2003).

Baby Boomers as a group hope that somehow aging will be different when they themselves become 65, 75, 85, and older. They see their grandparents and parents growing old and, though they may not articulate how aging should be different, they have a clear understanding that they do not want to grow old in the same way that those before them are growing old. Baby Boomers demand control over every phase of their lives and expect to control the aging process, to be in charge of their own health and health care and the manner of their deaths. In order to do this, they need to be assured that Social Security, Medicare, and Medicaid remain in place and viable for their future, and that they have the resources to keep them comfortably at home. Planning for old age needs to occur on both the individual and community levels (see Appendix [pp. 173–180] for a useful guide on individual planning).

As individuals, Baby Boomers generally ignore the fact of their own old age, opting to be seen as "forever young"—a defensive tactic that leads to little real forethought or planning for one's eighties and beyond. Our ageist attitudes have led our society to this state of mind in which we deny growing old in order not to be cast into a miserable existence of chronic ill health, poverty, and isolation. There is another way out of this as the Summit participants indicated. First, ill-health, depression, and poverty are not necessarily companions of old age and, in fact, each generation of older persons from the 1940s on have proven to be healthier, wealthier, and wiser than the preceding generation. Second, the Baby Boom generation holds in its power, through sheer numbers, the ability to create change to ensure that its eighties *CAN* be like its fifties, and for those who are experiencing hardships in their middle years, that old age *CAN* offer hope of a better life.

This can only happen if Baby Boomers become proactive and act now to initiate change.

Advocacy on the part of Baby Boomers and health care professionals, many of whom are also Baby Boomers, is the answer. The Baby Boom generation is perhaps the most diverse generation that the U.S. has ever produced. It is diverse in all respects—health, income, education, political leanings, lifestyles, culture, and country of birth. In spite of this, the generation can find common cause in a desire for an old age in which health and social care needs are met, income is sufficient, secure housing is available, and quality of life is good. But to realize this desire, action is needed now.

INCOME SECURITY

When they do look ahead to their old age, Baby Boomers focus on income security. The passing of the Social Security legislation in 1935 once meant that Americans could retire with confidence that having contributed to the federal social insurance program they would receive monthly income to support them for as long as they lived. This confidence has been eroded over the last 15 years. With rising costs and inflation, the Social Security check is no longer sufficient to enable retirees to maintain the same level of life style or even, for some, to keep them above the poverty level after they leave the workplace. Additional private savings, insurance coverage, pensions, and/or investments are necessary. Not all can afford to save for the future and, even for those who can, economic downturns and mismanagement of mutual funds and stocks and shares, as we have witnessed in the last few years, can traumatically decrease the value of an individual's holdings. Furthermore, the older population is expanding and life expectancy is increasing, thus placing pressures on the viability of the entire Social Security program over time.

The United States has been engaged in a discussion over the future of Social Security for many years but little has been done, except to raise the age for full eligibility from 65 to 67, in order to ensure that the program will remain strong throughout the twenty-first century. Baby Boomers are rightfully concerned, not only about Social Security but over the health insurance segments of Social Security—Medicare and Medicaid. Both these programs are seriously underfunded and are no longer able to make good on the country's original promise: to make comprehensive health care available to all older persons, regardless of income. Numerous changes have been made to Medicare, including the current administration's recent coverage of prescription drugs, but premiums and out-of-pocket costs continue to rise.

In the absence of a national health care insurance program, it is imperative that Medicare and Medicaid expand the health benefits that are covered and remain solvent in order to meet the needs of the current and future older populations. Baby Boomers wield clout due to their great numbers and could thus become a powerful and effective lobbying tool to ensure the continuation and strengthening of these programs. The recent Medicare legislation, although adding some coverage of prescription drugs, also adds to the profits of the pharmaceutical companies and health management organizations (HMOs), includes further cost-sharing on behalf of the beneficiaries, and appears to negate and place off limits the existing state-run programs that cover prescription drug costs, such as EPIC in New York State. The legislation is still too recent for the fine details or the real impact, negative and positive, to be fully understood, although there are advocates who have already placed Congress on notice that attempts will be made to alter or overrule it. Neither Medicare nor Medicaid should be allowed to become a partisan political battlefield. For the physical and mental health of the U.S. population, Medicare and Medicaid must continue to be accepted as entitlements for older persons and low income disabled populations. Furthermore, both programs need to provide extended coverage that includes not only prescription drugs, but medical equipment, assistive devices such as hearing aids and eyeglasses, preventive health care, and comprehensive coverage of health care in the community.

Action Steps for Baby Boomers

Save for retirement. If possible, invest in individual retirement accounts, add to workplace pension programs, and put money aside for the future.

Raise the issues. Encourage and engage in open discussion of the range of projections for "tomorrow." Explore your own financial means and expectations.

Advocate for needed changes to the federal programs and elect legislators who will make the changes happen. There is much debate and many diverse perspectives and solutions on how to "save" Social Security and what to do about health insurance, depending on each individual's political ideology. It is not the intent of the authors or the summit participants to support one solution over another but to challenge Baby Boomers to become involved and push to have the issues faced and rational and equable (not politically motivated), changes made.

Action Steps for Health and Social Service Professionals

All of the above and:

Educate and assist with applications for Medicaid, Supplementary Security Income (SSI), and health insurance programs.

Advocate. Develop community forums, discuss the issues, testify.

Collect data. Use service data and case experiences to illustrate the impact of current federal programs and the need for changes.

Involve the media.

HEALTH

Reaching and living through our later years in good health is largely dependent on our ability to practice a healthy lifestyle throughout our lives. Age-related diseases may be avoided or their effects minimized through lifelong habits of exercise, proper nutrition, safety precautions, management of stress, use of alcohol in moderation, and the avoidance of smoking. Although few would argue with this premise, changing behavior is a major undertaking and for the current older population and the frontrunners of the Baby Boomers, much of this knowledge was recognized too late to prevent uninformed lifestyle habits from taking root.

Individual healthy behavior is insufficient in itself. We also require maintenance of a healthy environment, free of toxins and pollution. Carbon emission and its impact on global warming, the maximization of profits over cleanup of industrial waste, and the continued decimation of our forests and open spaces all lead to compromised health for the individual and increasing frailty in old age for society as a whole.

All of us, not just the Baby Boomers, need to act, on the individual front by following healthy lifestyles, and in the public arena by advocating for a livable, healthy environment. This means publicizing environmental problems, supporting those legislators who are environmentally concerned, advocating for legislation where needed, and demanding a healthy world in which to live. Maintaining healthy lifestyles and promoting clean environments will benefit the nation as a whole.

However, even if we were able to effect all these changes, some degree of frailty and age-related disease would remain. Even with the increasing discoveries of genetic causal factors for age-related disease and our ongoing technological advances, chronic illness and living in old age with poor health are likely to remain in the future for some, regardless of whether they espouse healthy lifestyle behaviors. Older persons suffering from age-related diseases or chronic debilitating health conditions should never be considered responsible for their own frailty. In the past, ageist attitudes supported a tendency to blame the victim, denigrating old age and particularly the chronically ill.

Currently, older patients are discriminated against in the quality and level of health care they receive. A scarcity of health care professionals trained in care of the old and the continuing practice of ageist attitudes result in older persons often being denied the kind of preventive care routinely provided to others (Pope, 2003). A recent report by The Alliance for Aging Research noted that older persons are less likely than younger persons to be screened for diseases and tend to be undertreated for those diseases that are diagnosed (Alliance for Aging Research, 2003). Health care professionals as well as the general public tend to subscribe to ageist beliefs. Baby Boomers can be a powerful force in changing these beliefs by demanding health care treatment as they age that is equal to that provided to younger patients.

Action Steps for Baby Boomers

Exercise. Even if an individual has never engaged in exercise as part of a regular routine, advantages are gained from initiating regular exercise at any age.

Nutrition. Follow the guidelines for a healthy, balanced diet. Avoid fatty foods; include fruit, vegetables, and fiber foods.

Weight control. If over- or underweight, take steps to reach the advised weight for one's age and height.

Smoking and substance abuse. Join support groups and ask for assistance from health care professionals in changing these behaviors.

Safety. Take safety precautions such as use of seat belts, protection from the sun, smoke alarms in the home.

Stress management. Life in the U.S. can be stressful. Find ways that help you to minimize stress in your life and to deal with it when it occurs.

Environmental advocacy. Avoid individual pollution of our environment and support action on the local, state, and federal levels that make our environment healthy and safe.

Partner in health care. Take charge of your health care. Be an active partner with your health care professionals in demanding appropriate care equal to that received by younger patients. Seek out health care professionals with geriatric training. Join community health boards and local groups to advocate against ageism and for quality, integrated health care.

Action Steps for Health and Social Service Professionals

All of the above plus:

Education. Provide literature, give community presentations, advise clients and patients on the value of following healthy lifestyles. Educate about normal aging versus age-related health conditions.

Age discrimination. Review your practice and delivery of health or social service care for ageism. Abandon myths and change beliefs as indicated.

Programming. Establish exercise clubs, weight loss programs, community cleanup days, self-help groups, and so forth.

Advocacy. Join Baby Boomers in coalitions to testify, lobby, network, and vote.

LONG-TERM CARE

Long-term care, which incorporates health education and health maintenance as well as the monitoring and management of chronic health conditions, age-related diseases, and resulting functional deficits, is and will continue to be the heart of the health care system for older persons as well as younger persons with lifelong, chronic health issues. It is the structure and emphasis of our health care system, which is still locked into an acute care mode with its emphasis on immediate, hospital-based intervention and cure, that is in need of change. The growing emphasis on end-of-life care in the past few years is one area in which our health care system is beginning to recognize long-term care needs and a patient's right to involvement in care decisions. This shift in perspective needs to be extended. The health care system must play "catch up" with reality to become more relevant to today's and tomorrow's health care needs and expectations. It will require a shift in philosophies, outlooks, organizing, and financing structures, none of which will be easy to accomplish. Policy makers, administrators, educators, and health care practitioners all recognize that changes are required and there are promising models throughout the country but, to date, no one element or interest group has taken responsibility for dealing with the need to revise our health care system. Planning at national and local levels that includes representatives of all interested parties, and implementation that is carried out at the local level will allow us to overcome current fragmentation of health services and disparities between populations; to focus care within the community; and to position the patient and family as equal partners with health and social service providers in the development and management of care plans.

Federal legislation, in the form of the Olmstead Act, is promoting long-term care in the community as the preferred alternative to institutionalization. In order for this to be possible and effective, the needed health and social services must be made available at the local level. The development and increase in coordinated local services will place increasing importance on uniform standards, regulations, and procedural rules. Many of our existing health and social service programs operate as quasi-private organizations and are either unregulated or poorly monitored and unlicensed. A sea change to community-based services and programs to facilitate long-term care in the community can, as has been demonstrated in the past, attract the unscrupulous as well as the honest, and it will be imperative to establish appropriate guidelines and quality standards from the outset.

Cost of long term-care, whether in the community, as is the preferred goal, or in institutions such as nursing and mental health facilities, is prohibitive for all but the wealthy or those who have been able to purchase insurance coverage. Emphasis on care in the community and in the home environment can become a thinly veiled means of shifting costs from government (Medicaid) to the individual, but whether this occurs or not, care over a long period of time is costly and can quickly result in the impoverishment of the individual/family and a return of the costs to government under the existing Medicaid regulations. In the absence of a comprehensive federal health care insurance program, insurance companies are offering long-term care insurance. The plans are many and varied. In essence, until a majority of the adult population purchases such insurance at a young age, the premiums will remain relatively high. For many, the current cost may outweigh the calculated risk of needing long-term care in later years. Recent White House suggestions that long-term care premiums be tax deductible may be a help to some but may not encourage increased purchase of such insurance by those most likely to require this care—those in the lower income brackets—without government assistance. There are a few creative programs between government and the insurance companies, such as New York State's Partnership program, which has somewhat lowered premiums but which includes the intent to safeguard an individual's financial holdings. This feature has encouraged more persons to purchase long-term care insurance, thus guaranteeing that future care needs will be met while reducing government's responsibility.

Action Steps for Baby Boomers

Initiate and/or join community coalitions on behalf of integrated, long-term care in your community. Be a voice in establishing guidelines, promoting integration, demanding quality care that will be available to you if you need long-term care in your old age.

Collaborate with representatives of health and social services for the younger disabled and lower income populations to create a united voice.

Advocate for creative financing of long-term care costs.

Utilize advance directives to identify your preferences for end-of-life care.

Action Steps for Health and Social Service Professionals

All of the above plus:

Dialogue with Baby Boomers, listening to their needs and expectations for long-term care in the community. Include Baby Boomers as members of planning groups and Boards.

Educate members of your discipline in the care of older persons and the new skills and knowledge required by long-term care in the community.

Gain and promote knowledge and skills in providing end-of-life care.

Demand that the required skills and knowledge be imbedded in the curriculum of the professional, discipline-based schools.

Promote interest among students in specializing in care of older persons.

Continue to be or become a member of an interdisciplinary health care team.

LIFESTYLES AND ROLES

Society is already accepting of the changing and expanding lifestyles open to older persons and the numerous roles that they fill, whether by choice or circumstances. Full retirement from the work force, part-time work, acquiring new knowledge, exploring the world, volunteering, consultancy, new careers, self-employment, transmuting individual interests and skills into productive ventures, raising grandchildren, building second families, are all possibilities. Accompanying these varied lifestyles is a diversity of expanding roles—nurturer, leader, mentor, advisor, traveler, creator, activist, recorder, builder, sage. The currently diverse older population will become even more so as the Baby Boomers enter old age, and is expected to result in an equal expansion and growing diversity of lifestyles and roles.

In an ideal world, individuals would have a choice of the lifestyle and roles they experience and fill. In reality, income, health, location, life circumstances, and personality can either provide freedom of choice or conspire to limit an individual's options. The task for society is surely to level the playing field of old age, enabling older persons greater freedom in choosing between work and non-work and the various roles they fill.

Action Steps for Baby Boomers

Plan for old age and the lifestyle/roles you desire. This might take the form of learning a new skill, saving and budgeting, building relationships, changing habits, researching new locations.

Help build and belong to supportive networks of family, friends, and neighbors.

Engage in activities; become connected to the wider community.

Action Steps for Health and Social Service Professionals

All the above and:

Advocate for the elimination of poverty and the availability of quality health care for all.

Include older persons and members of the Baby Boom generation in the planning and oversight of the health and social service programs for which you are responsible.

Offer workshops on planning for old age; establish self-help groups.

LIVING ARRANGEMENTS

Living arrangements—where one lives, in what type of building, alone or with others, in city or country—play a crucial role in defining the quality of life in old age, and even more so for those living in poor health or with restricted mobility. Where one resides and in what kind of housing is therefore a crucial factor in planning for one's later years.

Where to live when one leaves the work force has long been part of planning for retirement for those in the middle income brackets. For some, this planning takes the form of investing in a vacation home with a view to its becoming the year-round residence in old age. For others, the careful research and visiting of likely places for retirement take on the aspects of selecting a college for their children. But even this careful forethought frequently fails to consider the possibility of a frail old age. For example, whereas the northeastern states may experience out-migrations of young retirees to the warmer states, there is often a reverse migration back when the younger retirees enter their eighties and require the proximity of their families and an increase in services. However, the majority of persons nearing retirement are not able to afford the luxury of determining where they will move, and many are more concerned with how they will be able to continue to afford their current housing.

For those older persons who wish to remain in their homes and communities where they have aged, ways need to be found to assure that the costs of remaining in place continue to be affordable and that environmental changes are made where necessary to accommodate potential frailty and long-term care needs for services. Government assistance in meeting utility costs, home sharing, and reverse mortgages are some of the existing programs that may help older persons meet their housing costs. Household renovations/repair programs and collaborative service efforts in communities designated as naturally occurring retirement communities (NORCs) are programs that enable older persons to remain in their homes.

For those older persons who do plan to move as they age, there are numerous types of living arrangements from which to choose, but the issue for most is not so much a lack of variety but a lack of affordable housing in many parts of the United States. Low-income housing is in short supply in most major cities, and although there is a modest expansion in the development of assisted living communities and senior housing, this is generally targeted to those with upper-middle incomes. There is thus a clear need for public/private partnerships to increase the stock of low-income housing and ensure that Baby Boomers will be able to secure affordable, gero-friendly housing as they age.

Action Steps for Baby Boomers

Consider options and plan for future good health and for the possibility of frailty.

Plan ahead to ensure that you will live in housing that provides a gero-friendly and safe environment for yourself in good health and will also be able to accommodate you if you become disabled. This might include seeking new housing, seeking others with whom to house partner, remodeling a current home, acquiring gero-safety devices, or radically changing current living arrangements, such as a move to sheltered housing, a senior residence, and so on.

Become involved in community action to make your community friendly to both well and disabled older persons. This might include increased public transportation; increased cultural, educational, and recreational facilities; large signage; ramped curbs; wider doorway access for mobility aids; intergenerational activities; or development of community parks.

Advocate for recognition of your immediate locality as a Naturally Occurring Retirement Community (NORC), if it qualifies. This could increase access to benefits and services.

Action Steps for Health and Social Service Professionals

All the above and:

Engage in community coalition building to establish recognized Naturally Occurring Retirement Communities where applicable.

Lobby and advocate for low-income senior housing.

Educate clients and patients on developing safe, secure environments in the home and promote gero-friendly design of new buildings.

HEALTH CARE PROFESSIONALS

The issues for health care professionals are clear. There are insufficient persons in all health care disciplines with geriatric/gerontological knowledge and skills to meet the health and social service needs of our current older population. The increasing numbers of aged in our near future will only mean that the gap between supply and demand will continue to grow. There is an urgent need for geriatric/gerontological training for those professionals already in practice as well as a focus on care of older persons within the professional schools, to ensure that all students graduate with some knowledge of aging. Parallel to this effort, there needs to be a shift in perspective within the professional schools about what curriculum is needed to prepare physicians, nurses, social workers, and all other health care disciplines to meet the realities of our changing health care system. "Like other health professions, social work is being compelled to rethink its mission and to identify the practice components needing change" (Pecukonis, Cornelius, & Parrish, 2003). Care in the community, long-term care, interdisciplinary teamwork, and other emerging trends all demand new curriculum content and, often, new ways of delivering services. Health care professionals and educators, many of whom are themselves Baby Boomers, need to reach out to Baby Boomers. The two groups need to listen to each other, to understand their needs and expectations, and recognize the potential limitations of existing resources.

Action Steps for Baby Boomers

Demand geriatric expertise from those caring for older family members now and for yourself when reaching old age.

Seek second opinions if your primary health care provider lacks geriatric expertise.

Action Steps for Health and Social Service Providers and Educators

Listen to the Baby Boomers. Health care professionals, many of whom are, themselves, Baby Boomers, need to join with Baby Boomers and hear each other's needs and expectations.

Increase your knowledge of aging. Participate in professional seminars and/or continuing education events on care of your older patients/clients.

Encourage your colleagues to do the same. Provide educational opportunities and lead seminars, grand rounds, lectures on aging and health care.

As educators, integrate aging content and the expectations of Baby Boomers into your classes.

As professional school administrators, offer specialization in geriatrics/gerontological studies and increase the number of students trained in geriatrics/gerontology.

TECHNOLOGY

The role of technology and the promise of future technological advances within all areas of life—housing, recreation, health, education, transportation, physical and mental activities—is rapidly changing lifestyles, the ways in which we interact, and individual and community environments. Planning for the future must include recognition of these possibilities and an appreciation of how technological advances may hinder or expedite the realization of the Baby Boomer's wishes for their future. Advances in knowledge and technology have contributed and continue to contribute to increased good health and longer life expectancy in the United States, and now technology is meeting needs and solving problems in ways that we recognize and in ways about which we can only guess. Technology already in use can

- revolutionize delivery of long-term care in the community, enabling health care professionals to make virtual house calls;

- enable the homebound to interact socially and functionally with the outside world;
- promote learning and expand the reach of educational institutions;
- connect large numbers of persons separated geographically into one community for a common purpose;
- provide opportunities, formerly out of reach, for recreation and cultural and social experiences;
- construct dwellings that maintain and "repair" themselves as needed;
- offer tools and devices that fulfill daily tasks; and more.

The action steps related to technology are the same for Baby Boomers and health and social service professionals. *Recognize them, embrace them* when they help goals to be reached, *demand new advances* as indicated, and *use them* to realize today's wishes for tomorrow.

Speakers at all three summit meetings repeated the common theme that if tomorrow's aging is to be realized as they would hope, it must come about through demand, collaboration, and unremitting advocacy. Participants and speakers alike agreed that society is experiencing great changes, and health care is in the process of being restructured. Individuals varied in their levels of pessimism or optimism as to the nature and impact of the changes but it was universally recognized that in order to make our eighties like our fifties, Baby Boomers and health and social service professionals must unite in advocacy and influence the changes. Baby Boomers have large numbers in their favor. This generation has never yet been ignored, and as it stands at the gateway to tomorrow, it is in an ideal position to shape the future in ways that will benefit not only the Baby Boomers but the generations to follow.

The purpose of the Summit meetings was to initiate dialogue, and the objective of this publication is to encourage, if not to command, active advocacy in all its forms.

REFERENCES

Alliance for Aging Research. *Ageism: How healthcare fails the elderly.* www.aging research.org/brochures/ageism/index.cfm.

Keegan, C., Gross, S., Fisher, I., & Remez, S. (2003). *Boomers at midlife: The AARP life stage study. Wave 2, 2003. Executive summary.* Washington, DC: PSRA International.

Pecukonis, E., Cornelius, L., & Parrish, M. (2003). The future of health social work. *Social Work in Health Care, 37*(3), 1–15.

Pope, E. (2003). Second-class care. *AARP Bulletin, 44*(10), 6–8.

Appendix

Reproduced by permission of Robyn Golden

Mapping Your Future

Ranking Your Responses

The knowledge you gain from exploring your options can make your life easier, less stressful and give you more control of your future. To help you find out more about the areas of your life which could benefit from additional planning, rank each of the five statements in sections A–J below in terms of how close it is to your own activities and thoughts about your life or planning.

In each section, use the number "5" to indicate the statement that is most important to you, or to which you most agree; the number "4" to indicate which statement is second most important to you, or to which you next most agree, and so forth, using the number "1" to indicate the statement least important to you, not like you, or to which you least agree.

Repeat the process until you complete all sections, A–J. Each section should have only one "5," one "4," one "3," one "2," and one "1" ranking.

Rank the five statements in EACH section from 5 to 1:

"5" = Most important to me
"4" = Second most important to me
"3" = Third most important to me
"2" = Fourth most important to me
"1" = Least important to me

A

_____ I visit my doctor at least once a year for checkups and tests.
_____ I actively participate in managing my financial affairs.

_____ I have family and/or friends who will help care for me in the future if I need it.

_____ I have lots of choices for working, volunteering, learning, or doing other things for myself.

_____ I have a good idea of where I want to live as I get older.

B

_____ A social life that occupies most of my time is very important to me.

_____ I have one or more hobbies that I pursue actively and plan to continue them.

_____ I've gotten my financial situation pretty well planned.

_____ I am concerned that some day I won't be able to drive.

_____ I've looked into other housing I might consider if I needed or wanted to move.

C

_____ My spiritual life plays an important role for me as I get older.

_____ It is hard for me to be confident that I'll have enough money in the future.

_____ I've identified some productive activities I can do as I get older.

_____ I've planned for my health needs in the future.

_____ I am concerned that some day I won't be able to live independently.

D

_____ I've planned for my own and my family's future financial needs.

_____ I know what it would take to move if I had to or wanted to.

_____ I've thought about the health challenges I think I will face as I get older.

_____ I have thought about who I could turn to for needed help in the future.

_____ I have found a way to fill my days with enjoyable things to do.

E

_____ I have made my wishes for my health care clear to my family or caregivers.

_____ It is hard for me to talk to my children/friends about the things I am concerned about.

_____ I've planned how to stay busy and productive as I get older.

_____ I've considered how to make my home easier and safer to live in.

_____ I have estimated how long I think I'll live and how much money I'll need.

F

_____ I am concerned that someday I'll have to live alone.

_____ My main concern about my future is that I will become ill and dependent.

_____ I am comfortable that I'll have family and friends to enjoy in the future.

_____ I'm concerned that without activities my spouse/partner and I will argue.

_____ I am concerned that I won't have enough money to maintain my current lifestyle.

G

_____ I am concerned that someday I'll have to sell my home and move somewhere else.

_____ I have the personal relationships that will be most important to me as I grow older.

_____ It is hard for me to talk to doctors about my health concerns.

_____ I'm concerned that I'll be bored in the future.

_____ I am concerned that I won't have enough money to pay for my medical expenses.

H

_____ I am concerned that in the future I won't be able to enjoy the activities I enjoy the most now.

_____ I am concerned that someday it won't be possible to live in my community or close to my friends.

_____ I have anticipated the health habits I'll have to adopt to stay healthy.

_____ I have a good place to live in my retirement.

_____ I have the income to maintain the lifestyle I'd like during my later years.

I

_____ I'm concerned that I may have to move from my home when I get older.

_____ I contact friends or local organizations when I'm looking for a new activity.

_____ I worry that I won't be able to afford to retire or will need a job for health insurance.

_____ Most of my current friends have been part of my life for a long time.

_____ I exercise regularly and watch my diet carefully to maintain my health and vigor.

J

_____ I am concerned that there will be no one to take care of me when I can no longer care for myself.

_____ I have done some planning such as making a will, trust, power of attorney, etc.

_____ There are things I do to maintain good mental health.

_____ I have a pretty good plan for how to keep active as I get older.

_____ I know what type of housing I'll live in as I get older.

Mapping Your Future

Recording Your Responses

Counting and Recording Your Score

Mapping Your Future reveals your planning and attention to five important life areas:

Health   Work and Leisure   Finances   Housing   Relationships

Each section box (A–J) has a statement corresponding to these five life areas. Be sure that you rate **each** statement on the Response pages. It is important to assign the numbers 1 through 5 within each of the section boxes (A–J). If you missed any, go back now and complete your responses.

Instructions:
1) Enter your scores for Sections A through J in the scoring box columns below.
2) After you've entered all the scores for each life area, add the numbers in each column and write the result in the line underneath the corresponding column.

Scoring Box

	Health	Work & Leisure	Finances	Housing	Relation-ships	
A						A
B						B
C						C
D						D
E						E
F						F
G						G
H						H
I						I
J						J

Total _____ + _____ + _____ + _____ + _____ = 150

Your score totals should add up to 150. Remember, each row should contain the numbers 1, 2, 3, 4, or 5 only once. If not, recheck that you have entered the individual scores correctly on the previous pages, transferred them to the scoring box accurately, and used each number only once within each section.

What do the scores mean?

40–50   These issues are important to you. You've either paid a lot of attention to anticipating your needs and the resources you'll need or it may be difficult for you to think about this area. Begin to concentrate on down-to-earth techniques for examining this area if it is troublesome or other life areas of Mapping Your Future if you're comfortable with the planning you have already done. Keep in mind that a balanced approach is the best way to plan for your future.

30–39   Although this area hasn't been your first priority, you've paid attention to these issues as a major aspect of what you know will be important to you in the future. Continue to update your needs and resources.

20–29   You've done a moderate amount of thinking and planning around this area. Continue to pay attention to these issues by assessing your needs and identifying the information and resources you'll need to feel confident that you've planned adequately.

10–19   This area is a low priority for you right now. You may have done quite a bit of planning already or it may raise issues that make you feel uncomfortable. It's important to remember that each of the life areas in Mapping Your Future requires consideration. This will enable you to best enjoy all aspects of your life.

Mapping Your Future

Planning Categories

Now That You've Taken Your Quiz

Aging is a process that no two people experience in the same way, at the same pace, or with the same assets and limitations and strengths. What we do have in common is that we want to age gracefully, in good health, and with few worries. What it means to age in our culture is changing dramatically.

Pre-planning, taking preventive measures, and attempting to anticipate future needs will put you in control of your own aging. Most life issues fall into the categories of health, work/leisure, finances, housing, and relationships. Try to anticipate what the issues facing you might be, when you may need help, and how you would want to resolve the challenges you might face. Taking these actions will allow you to enjoy your future years to the fullest.

Health relates to how you take care of your body, mind, and spirit. To many people, good mental and physical health is the greatest blessing that can be bestowed upon them. Because health affects all aspects of how you live and the quality of your life, it is no surprise that it is a concern to many. You can always take steps to help assure you will be happier and better able to enjoy your life in the future. Personal lifestyle choices, such as a healthy diet, regular exercise, and keeping active, are all important aspects. Remember, an ounce of prevention is worth a pound of cure. It is a smart idea to periodically evaluate your physical, mental, emotional, and spiritual strengths and weaknesses. You can assess anticipated needs and address your current and future abilities and disabilities. Planning can make a difference in how you manage possible changes.

If your lowest score is in the area of health, you may want to think about the following:

- Do you have access to affordable medical, social, and psychological health care?
- Do you try to follow your physician's health care recommendations?
- How often do you exercise?
- How is your diet? Do you try to eat a healthy, balanced diet geared to your age and health needs?
- Do you have a living will or written directives for health care interventions should you be unable to make your wishes known?

- How will you cope if you are affected by some of the more common health problems of aging—changes in vision, hearing loss, arthritis and joint pain, decline in physical strength, energy, and agility?
- Do your relationships need improvement?
- Do you find meaning through spirituality?
- Do you engage in mentally stimulating activities?
- Are your needs for sexual and emotional closeness being met?
- Do you often feel sad and alone?
- Do you try to expand your social and family contacts?

NEXT STEPS FOR MAPPING YOUR FUTURE

How do you want to spend your retirement? Traveling, volunteering, taking up a new interest, starting a new career? You can spend your retirement in style, but a lot of pieces go into creating the life you want.

By addressing your long-term financial needs, planning where you will live, organizing how you will spend your time, strengthening connections to family and friends, and protecting your health today, you may lead the life you're dreaming about tomorrow.

APPENDIX I:

SOCIAL WORK FELLOWS PLANNING COMMITTEE

Sonya Austrian
Barbara Brenner
Phyllis Caroff
Rose Dobrof
Zelda Foster
Natalie Gordon
Judith Howe
Myrna Lewis
Mildred Mailick
Helen Rehr
Patricia Volland

Nadine Gartrell, Staff

APPENDIX II: SUMMIT PRESENTERS

Ronald D. Adelman, MD, is Co-Chief of the Division of Geriatrics and Gerontology and an Associate Professor of Medicine at the Weill Medical College of Cornell University. He served on the faculty of the Columbia College of Physicians and Surgeons, Mount Sinai School of Medicine, and was the founding Division Chief of Geriatric Medicine at Winthrop University Hospital, a major affiliate of S.U.N.Y. Stony Brook School of Medicine. Dr. Adelman is also Director of the Cornell Center for Aging Research and Clinical Care (CARCC), a multidisciplinary group of scientists, clinicians, and educators who seek to speed scientific advances from bench to bedside, teach geriatric medicine to physicians-in-training at all levels, and create a trans-institutional community of gerontologists at Cornell. Dr. Adelman's major area of research interest is physician–older patient communication and its influence on health outcomes. He has published extensively and is the co-author of a major textbook on elder abuse and neglect.

Katherine Briar-Lawson, PhD, is Dean of the School of Social Welfare, University at Albany. Dr. Briar-Lawson is nationally recognized for her expertise in family-focused practice and child and family policy. She is co-author of *Family-Centered Policies and Practices: International Implications* (2001), and co-editor of *Innovative Practices with Vulnerable Children and Families* (2001), *Evaluation Research in Child Welfare* (2002), and *Charting the Impacts of University–Child Welfare Collaboration* (2003). Dr. Briar-Lawson is a member of the Council of Social Work Education (CSWE) Practice Commission, associate editor of *New Global Development: Journal of International and Comparative Social Welfare,* and consulting editor for *Social Work and Family Preservation.* She is co-chair of the Gerontological Task Force of the National Association for Deans and Directors.

Robert N. Butler, MD, is President, CEO, and Co-Chair of the Alliance for Health and the Future, of the International Longevity Center—USA. Dr. Butler is also Professor of Geriatrics at The Brookdale Department of Geriatrics and Adult Development at The Mount Sinai Medical Center, New York City. Dr. Butler was the founding Director of the National Institute on Aging of the National Institutes of Health and later founded the first Department of Geriatrics in a U.S. medical school at Mount Sinai School of Medicine, where he held the Brookdale Professorship of Geriatrics. More recently he co-founded the International Longevity Center (ILC), a policy, research, and education center with Centers in

France, the United Kingdom, the Dominican Republic, Japan, and the U.S. Dr. Butler won the Pulitzer Prize for his book *Why Survive? Being Old in America* and is co-author of the books *Aging and Mental Health* and *Love and Sex After 60. The Longevity Revolution* is in preparation. Dr. Butler was the Chair of the advisory committee for the 1995 White House Conference on Aging. He has received numerous awards, the most recent being the Heinz Award for the Human Condition.

Michael Diaz, MD, is an Assistant Clinical Professor of Medicine at Mount Sinai Medical Center. Dr. Diaz has been at Mount Sinai Medical Center (MSMC) since 1974, where he has served as Assistant Director of Medical Care Services, Clinic Chief of the International Hemophilia Training Center, and Regional Comprehensive Hemophilia Center, co-founder and Co-Chief of the Sickle Cell Clinic, Medical Director of the Emergency Room, and MSMC representative to the Health Systems Agency of New York City, District Board 5. He is a member of the Community Board of MSMC and has served as a member of the MSMC Rape Intervention Program. Dr. Diaz helped to establish multiple medical clinics in rural areas of the Dominican Republic and assisted in the development of a continuous education program and a quality assurance program in the Gulf and Western Medical Center at La Romana, D.R.

Mathy Mezey, EdD, RN, FAAN, is the Independence Foundation Professor of Nursing Education, Division of Nursing, Steinhardt School of Education at New York University, and Director of the John A. Hartford Foundation Institute for Geriatric Nursing. Formerly Dr. Mezey was a Professor at the University of Pennsylvania School of Nursing, where she directed the Geriatric Nurse Practitioner Program and the Robert Wood Johnson Foundation Teaching Nursing Home Program. Dr. Mezey has authored multiple publications. She is Editor for the Springer series in Geriatric Nursing and of the Springer publication *The Encyclopedia of Elder Care*. Dr. Mezey's current research and writing focus on quality of care of older persons in hospitals and long-term care.

John Rother, JD, is the Director of Policy and Strategy for AARP, responsible for the federal and state public policies of the Association, for international initiatives, and for formulating AARP's overall strategic plan. Mr. Rother formerly served 8 years with the U.S. Senate as Special Counsel for Labor and Health to Senator Jacob Javits (R-NY) and then as Staff Director and Chief Counsel for the Senate Special Committee on

Aging. Mr. Rother serves on several boards and commissions including Generations United, the National Health Care Quality Forum, the American Board of Internal Medicine Foundation, National Academy of Aging, and Civic Ventures. He is an authority on managed care, long-term care, Social Security, pensions, and the challenges facing the baby boom generation.

Donna A. Shalala, PhD, is Professor of Political Science and President of the University of Miami. Prior to this appointment, Dr. Shalala served as Assistant Secretary for Policy Research and Development at the Department of Housing and Urban Development (HUD); President of Hunter College, City University of New York; Secretary of the United States Department of Health and Human Services; and Chancellor of the University of Wisconsin-Madison. Dr. Shalala has been awarded more than 30 honorary degrees.

Bruce C. Vladeck, MD, is Professor of Health Policy and Geriatrics at Mount Sinai School of Medicine and a member of numerous social-health organizations. Dr. Vladeck was President of the United Hospital Fund in New York and Administrator of the Health Care Financing Administration (HCFA) of the U.S. Department of Health and Human Services. Subsequent to his service at HCFA, Dr. Vladeck was appointed by President Clinton to the National Bipartisan Commission on the Future of Medicare. Dr. Vladeck was elected to the Institute of Medicine's (IOM) National Academy of Sciences and has chaired its Committee on Health Care for Homeless People. Among many honors and awards, Dr. Vladeck received the IOM's 1995 National Public Service Award, the 1996 Hubert H. Humphrey Award of the American Political Science Association, and the 1998 President's Award of the American Society on Aging. Dr. Vladeck is a nationally recognized expert on health care policy, health care financing, and long-term care. His many publications include *Unloving Care: The Nursing Home Tragedy* (Basic Books, 1980).

APPENDIX III:

WORKSHOP LEADERS AND REPORTERS

Summit Meetings 10/01; 4/02; 10/02

Jacquelin Berman
Denise Burnette
Suleika Cabrera-Drinane
Gina Cantenucci
Carol Capello
Li-Mei Chen
Nadine Cou
Judy Dobrof
Deidre Downs
Helene Ebenstein
Pat Gilberto
Roberta Graziano
Judith Howe
Evelyn Laureano
Myrna Lewis
Monica Matthiew
Edwin Méndez-Santiago
Clarener Moultrie
Nora O'Brien
James O'Neal
Anne O'Sullivan
Eliza Rossman
Danylle Rudin
Andrea Sherman
Renee Solomon
Maria Vezina
Cynthia Wagner
Brad Zodikoff

Index

Action steps
    financial security, 161–62
    health care professionals, 162, 164,
        166–67, 168
    healthy behaviors, 163–64, 167–68
Activities of Daily Living (ADLs), 61
Advance care planning, 77–82
African Americans, 13–19
Agent selection, 79
Age-related diseases, 60
AIDS, 13–14
Alternative medicine, 11–12
    See also Holistic approach
Anti-aging movement, 88–90
Assisted living, 104–5

Baby boomers
    action steps for, 161–62, 163–64,
        166, 167–68, 169, 170–71
    beliefs and concerns, 4–5, 27–34
    current situation, 3, 10–12
    future of, 21–24
    statistics, 9
    See also Summit Series
Biogerontologists, 90
Bush Administration
    proposed Medicare changes, 50
Butler, Robert N., 50–51

Cancer, 13–14
Cardiovascular disease, 13–14
Caregivers, 63–68

family, 63–67
    formal, 67–68
Case studies, 107–109
Celebrities, 32–33
Childbearing, 28–29
Chronic conditions, 22, 61–62
    disparities, 13–14, 20
Clinton Administration
    proposed Medicare changes, 49
Cohort phenomenon, 38
Communities
    action readiness, 156
    defined, 154
    living in, 99–103
    long-term care and, 70–72, 165–66
    mobilization capacity, 155
    services, 102–3
    See also Naturally Occurring Retire-
        ment Communities (NORCs)
Community collaboration, 148–57
    about, 148–51
    building, 153–57
    models of, 151–52
Congregate housing, 104
Consumer Reports, 69–70
Cultural issues, 16, 18
    caregiving, 65
Current trends
    geriatrics, 123–24, 127–28
    health care delivery, 146–48
    health insurance, 53–54
    living arrangements, 97–99

Current trends *(continued)*
  Medicare, 20–21
  nursing homes, 21

Death, 79–80
  See also End-of-life care
Diabetes, 13–14, 55
Disability rates, 62
Discrimination, 16–19
Disparities
  health, 12–19
  income, 23, 44–45
Documenting preferences, 79
Downsizing living arrangements,
    100–101
Drugs, 22, 29–30

Economics of long-term care, 64,
    68–70
Educated consumers, 57–58
Education
  continuing, 93, 118
  of health care professionals, 56–57,
    128–42
Employer-based medical insurance,
    53–54
End-of-life care, 33–34, 74–82
  advance care planning, 77–80
  changes in, 74–76
  palliative care, 76–77
Environmental issues, 18–19

Family structure, 39–40, 66–67
Financial resources
  disparities, 15
  predictions, 39
Financial security
  action steps, 161–62
Fitness, 31

Genetic decoding, 31
Geriatrics, 123–44
  current model, 123–24, 127–28
  emergent trends, 126–27
  holistic approach, 125–26
  nursing education, 128–30

physician education, 136–42
social work education, 130–36

Health care delivery, 46–59
  current trends, 146–48
  improvement areas, 17–18
  NORC-SSP services, 117–18
  quality of, 14–15
  See also Holistic approach; Medicare
Health care professionals, 127–28,
    170–71
  action steps for, 162, 164, 166–67,
    168, 170, 171
  nurses, 128–30
  physicians, 136–42
  social workers, 130–36
Health insurance. *See* Insurance
Healthy behaviors
  action steps for, 162–64
  disparities, 18
  See also Lifestyles; Summit Series
Hispanics, 13–19
HMOs, 50, 54
Holistic approach, 125–26, 129–30,
    135–43
Home care, 64–65, 70–71, 102–3
Hospice, 77
Housing. *See* Living arrangements

IADLs, 61–62
Income
  disparities, 23
  security, 35–45, 160–62
Independent senior housing, 102
Infant mortality
  disparities, 13–14
Institutional living, 103–6
Instrumental Activities of Daily Living.
    See IADLs
Insurance, 46–47
  current trends, 53–54
  disparities, 15–16
  long-term care, 69–70
  the uninsured, 49
Interdisciplinary team approach,
    125–26

Kevorkian, Jack, 75
401 (k)s, 42–43

Lifestyles, 23–24, 62–63, 90–94
  action steps, 167–68
Living arrangements, 23–24, 97–110,
    168–70
  action steps, 169
  community, 99–103
  current status, 97–99
  institutional, 103–6
Living wills, 81
Long-term care, 55–56, 60–73, 164–67
  action steps for, 166–67
  caregivers, 63–68
  communities, 165–66
  consumer involvement, 70–72
  financing, 68–70

Marketing to retirees, 93
Medicaid, 51–52
  and long-term care, 68–70
Medical power of attorney, 81
Medicare
  background, 47–48
  current state of, 20–21
  disparities, 15–16
  future of, 49–51
  and long-term care, 68–70
  recent changes, 48–49
Medicine
  advances in, 20
Menopause, 30
Minorities
  health disparities, 12–19

National Center for Minority Health
    and Health Disparities (NIH),
    16–17
Naturally Occurring Retirement Com-
    munities (NORCs), 99–100,
    111–13
NORC-Supportive Service programs
    (NORC-SSP), 113–22
  about, 113–17
  future of, 120–21

lessons learned, 119–20
New York participation, 115–16
services, 117–19
Nursing education, 128–30
Nursing homes, 14–15, 21, 106

Obesity, 32, 54–55

Palliative care, 76–77
Physical activity programs, 55
Physician education, 136–42
Planning Ahead, 78–80
Plastic surgery, 33
Politics, 28
Power of attorney, medical, 81
Preventive activities, 147
  See also Holistic approach

Quality of life. See Lifestyles

Recreation, 118
Rent subsidies, 102
Research, 56
Rethinking, 80
Retirement, 23, 84–96
  Baby Boomers and, 87–88
  changes in perspective, 40–42, 84–85
  communities, 101
  lifestyles, 90–94
  work after, 43–45, 85–87
Right to Die movement, 34
Rother, John, 50

Senior centers, 93–94
Seniors today, statistics, 8–9
Sexual revolution, 28
Shalala, D, 58
Shared-living residences, 101–2
Social isolation, 92
Social Security
  future of, 36–38, 40–43
  private sector investments in, 42
Social work
  education, 130–36
  services, 117
Successful aging, 95

Summit Series, 1–3, 6–7
  recommendations, 158–72
SUPPORT Principal Investigators, 76

Technology, 171–72
"Third Rail," 58

Universal design homes, 106

Viagra, 30
Vladeck, B., 40, 41, 58
Volunteerism, 94, 118

Women
  of color, 17
  and Social Security, 44
Work
  after retirement, 43–45
  patterns, 23
World view, 38–39

Springer Series on Life Styles and Issues in Aging

Bernard D. Starr, PhD, Series Editor
Marymount Manhattan College, New York, NY

Advisory Board: Robert C. Atchley, PhD; Marjorie Cantor, PhD (Hon); Harvey L. Sterns, PhD

2005   **Baby Boomers: Can My Eighties Be Like My Fifties?**
M. Joanna Mellor, DSW, and Helen Rehr, DSW, DSc(Hon)

2005   **Community Care for an Aging Society: Issues, Policies, and Services**
Carole B. Cox, PhD

2003   **Women in the Middle: Their Parent-Care Years, 2nd Edition**
Elaine M. Brody, MSW, DSc(Hon)

2003   **Successful Aging and Adaptation With Chronic Diseases**
Edited by Leonard W. Poon, PhD, Phil, hc, Sarah Hall Gueldner, DSN, FAAN, and Betsy M. Sprouse, PhD

2000   **Elders, Crime, and the Criminal Justice System: Myth, Perceptions, and Reality in the 21st Century**
Edited by Max B. Rothman, JD, LLM, Burton D. Dunlop, PhD, and Pamela Entzel, JD

2000   **Empowering Grandparents Raising Grandchildren: A Training Manual for Group Leaders**
Carole B. Cox, PhD

1999   **To Grandmother's House We Go and Stay: Perspectives on Custodial Grandparents**
Edited by Carole B. Cox, PhD

1999   **Preservation of the Self in the Oldest Years: With Implications for Practice**
Sheldon S. Tobin, PhD

1998   **Working with Toxic Older Adults: A Guide to Coping with Difficult Elders**
Gloria M. Davenport, PhD

1998   **Ethnogerocounseling: Counseling Ethnic Elders and Their Families**
Virginia S. Burlingame, PhD

1997   **Life Beyond 85 Years: The Aura of Survivorship**
Colleen L. Johnson, PhD, and Barbara M. Barer, MSW

1995   **Gerocounseling: Counseling Elders and Their Families**
Virginia S. Burlingame, MSW, PhD

1995   **Impact of Increased Life Expectancy: Beyond the Gray Horizon**
Mildred M. Seltzer, PhD

1994   **Aging and Quality of Life**
Ronald P. Abeles, PhD, Helen C. Gift, PhD, and Marcia G. Ory, PhD, MPH

1993   **Retirement Counseling: A Handbook for Gerontology Practitioners**
Virginia E. Richardson, PhD

Springer Publishing Company

Community Care for an Aging Society

Issues, Policies, and Services

Carole B. Cox, PhD

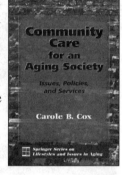

Most older persons desire to remain living in the community, but those requiring care are often at risk of not having their needs met. Families may find themselves unable to care for their older relatives, while formal services are often unavailable or inaccessible. Policies and services are beginning to focus on the community rather than institutions as the primary axis for care.

This book examines the many factors contributing to needs for care among older persons as well as the ways in which impairments are defined and responded to by both the individual and society. Focusing on practice and policy issues, Dr. Cox describes many of the early stage community care innovations that hold the promise of making contributions to the well-being and independence of the older population.

The scope of the book makes it appropriate for students in gerontology, public policy, social work, and sociology. In addition, the book has practical application for planners and service providers.

Contents:
- Community Care for an Aging Population
- Determining Needs for Care
- Policy and Care
- Community Programs and Services
- Housing Needs and Responses
- The Role of the Family in Providing Care
- Ethnicity and Care
- New Responses in Community Care
- The Challenges of Care for an Aging Population

Lifestyles and Issues in Aging Series
2005   192pp   0-8261-2804-1   hardcover

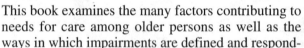

11 West 42nd Street, New York, NY 10036-8002 • Fax: 212-941-7842
Order Toll-Free: 877-687-7476 • Order On-Line: www.springerpub.com